The Samaritans: Befriending the suici

The Samaritans:

Befriending the suicidal

Edited and with an Introduction by

CHAD VARAH

Constable London

First published in Great Britain 1985
by Constable and Company Limited
10 Orange Street London WC2H 7EG

Revised edition 1987

Set in Linotron Bembo 11pt by
Rowland Phototypesetting Ltd
Bury St Edmunds, Suffolk
Printed in Great Britain by
St Edmundsbury Press Ltd
Bury St Edmunds, Suffolk

British Library CIP data
The Samaritans: befriending the suicidal –
Rev. ed.
1. Samaritans (*Organization*) – History
I. Varah, Chad
362.2 HV6548.G7

ISBN 0 09 467780 8

'The men and women of Melphé, the mere run of mankind,' said the King, 'it is they whom we have to consider first, and their poor human needs. It takes so very little to content them. They need only a home and food, a little work, their mates and their children. Out of these simple things, in the ever-present black shadow of chance and death, they create, very incredibly, their content. So for their sake, Cesario, you must now put aside Branlon, and the fine dreams of your youth, and your rights as a private person to any special happiness . . . If you do not take the throne when Lorenzo dies, then there is none to inherit . . . All would drift back . . . into the bleak bright savagery of Duke Sigismond's time: and my Melphé would be destroyed . . .'

'I created Melphé. I cannot make phrases about it, Cesario: but in that great red and grey and green, quiet city, where now some two hundred shops have just put up their shutters for the night, and where in the plaza the town band are tuning their instruments at this very instant, there, during Sigismond's black time, were untilled fields and burned huts and frightened people living desperately upon what they could take by blind force from one another. Now, in place of those naked mudflats, at Sinapoli is a prospering seaport; and back of it are Melphé and Pania and Ferata, all blended into one kingdom . . .

'To help human beings some little way towards orderly and contented living, is that not a dream as brave and strange as is any dream of Branlon? That is what I have done, Cesario, here in my little Melphé, in my own commonplace and prosaic decreed kingdom. I have worked with what tools I might, with Holy Church and your mother's whoredoms, with Sacrobosco the assassin and with the town band . . . I have worked always in the service of my dream, of my own small, unimaginative, sane dream. It has been made tangible through my long labours. Now it is threatened . . . Cesario, my staid strong dream must not perish now that I go down, so very feebly, to my last sleep, beyond the reach of all human dreams!'

'My father,' said Cesario, 'it shall not perish! I have given men songs where you gave them sewerage . . . While my songs were but so-so, your sewers were of the first order. I must see to it that they are kept in sound condition . . .'

The King said then: 'Pardon my loquaciousness. In one more moment I shall rest . . . The Spanish are so improvident as to raise merino wool for us, and then to buy back at our own prices, mind you, the cloths we make out of it. So their wools ought to be admitted duty free. Do you remember, Cesario, as my last word to you, now that I die, there should be no further tariff upon the Spanish wools. Then, too, in regard to the allied matter of their wines –'

With that, the old gentleman paused, as if somewhat surprised. His lips parted. You saw he was trying to moisten them, and could not quite manage it.

'But this,' he said, in aggrieved protest against the intrusiveness of death, 'this is important. In regard to the customs duties upon Spanish wines –'

He breathed sighingly, as if acquiescent, at last, in his own defeat; and his large grey head fell sideways a little, towards the left. He lifted it, though, rigidly, with an effort very painful to witness; and then lay back, prosaic and grotesque, but erect, in his tall chair, facing the sunset . . .

Hermia slipped from off her finger the ring containing the bezoar stone. It had not ever left her finger since Cesario placed it there upon the beach at Gratignolles. To remove it was the one thing which she had refused to old Ferdinand during his lifetime. She removed it now. She gave back the ring to him who had first placed it upon her finger, reaching out to him over the dead body of her husband.

From *The king was in his counting-house*, JAMES BRANCH CABELL

Foreword

The Samaritans: Befriending the Suicidal (2nd edition) is the 1987 version of the book *The Samaritans* which I prepared for our twelfth anniversary in 1965. The book was updated as *The Samaritans in the 70s* for our twentieth anniversary in 1973, and when this was revised in 1977 about one-third of the material in it was replaced or rewritten.

In 1980 I rewrote the introduction to answer the questions people were still asking after reading the previous books, and replaced most of the previous material except for the greater part of the section on Depression, which in my view could not be, or at any rate has not been, bettered. *The Samaritans in the 80s* (1980) was thus substantially a new book.

Another revision was needed in 1984, because the enormous expansion of our work especially outside the British Isles rendered the list of Branches incomplete and sometimes inaccurate. Every list becomes out of date even whilst it is being printed, but when lives may depend upon people being able to find our centres, we have a duty to be as accurate as we can, hoping that if one centre is unavailable another not far away may be approached.

The Samaritans: Befriending the Suicidal retains the section on Crisis, Depression and Anxiety, but most of the remaining material has been rewritten or replaced. The book was again revised in 1986 and the list of our Branches all over the world updated to October 1986. The outstanding addition to the text is *Ten Commonalities of Suicide* by probably the world's leading suicidologist, Edwin S. Shneidman, which I have placed immediately after our seven Principles and Practices. His no. 5 expresses with admirable lucidity why The Samaritans and his own colleagues in the AAS are responding rightly and most other services wrongly: 'It is neither possible nor practical in an individual who is highly lethal and highly perturbed to attempt to deal with the lethality directly.' This confirms my own 'The person in crisis is too fragile to have his problems tackled. We must first befriend the person who has the problems.'

In 1978 the movement presented me with a *Festschrift* entitled *Answers to suicide, presented to Chad Varah by The Samaritans on the 25th anniversary of their founding* (Constable £2.95), answering twenty questions I had been invited to pose. The answer to my ninth question, 'What kind of attention does a person need who has been medically rescued after an act of self-injury?' by Professor Ivor Mills is reprinted here under the title 'Befriending those who cannot cope'. Also reprinted from the same book is Dominique Alessandri's indispensable article 'How can Samaritans be protected from useless manipulation by the psychopath?' I hope these will lead people to read the whole book.

Many Branch and other libraries retain the earlier versions of this present book. Apart from my Introduction in its different forms, readers may wish to look up some excellent articles not reprinted here. For the sake of the new generation of Samaritans, I have reprinted the essay on Psychological Problems by our late beloved President, Dr Doris Odlum, contributed to the 1965 edition, and still instructive in her inimitable way.

CHAD VARAH
London, October 1986

Contents

I saw one fallen in the sand, half sitting, half lying upon his hands. This was a religious mendicant, some miserable derwish in his clouted beggar's cloak, who groaned in extremity, holding forth his hands like eagles' claws to man's pity. Last in the long train, we went also marching by him. His beggar's scrip, full of broken morsels, fallen from his neck, was poured out before him. The wretch lamented to the slow moving lines of the Mecca-bound pilgrimage: the many had passed on, and doubtless as they saw his dying, hoped inwardly the like evil ending might not be their own. Some charitable serving men, Damascenes, in our company stepped aside to him; *ana meyet*, sobbed the derwish, I am a dying man. One then of our crew, he was also my servant, a valiant outlaw, no holy-tongue man but of human deeds, with a manly heartening word, couched by an empty camel, and with a spring of his stalwart arms, lifted and set him fairly upon the pack saddle. The dying derwish gave a weak cry much like a child, and hastily they raised the camel under him and gathered his bag of scattered victuals and reached it to him, who sat all feeble murmuring thankfulness, and trembling yet for fear. There is no ambulance service with the barbarous pilgrim army; and all charity is cold, in the great and terrible wilderness, of that wayworn suffering multitude.

From *Travels in Arabia Deserta* Vol 1, p 91,
by Charles M. Doughty
(Constable & Co)

Introduction – CHAD VARAH

'What gave you the idea?'

For over thirty years people have been asking me this within a few minutes of meeting me. If there had been a simple answer, I should soon have got sick of hearing myself repeat it. But any answer attempting to be accurate would be far too long for a dinner table conversation or an interview with a journalist, let alone a television appearance where one may be required to deal with half a dozen questions in two and a quarter minutes; as will be evident when I try to explain the origin and ethos of The Samaritans in the following pages.

Years of attempting to reduce the length and complexity of the answer without distorting the facts have produced the following.

For as long as I can remember I have been a scientist, i.e. a person with a persistent curiosity about how and why, preferring facts to opinions and experiment to guesswork. So when I read in 1953 that there were three suicides a day in London, my restless mind busied itself with the question 'Why?'

I knew nothing about suicide and unthinkingly accepted the view then prevalent that you had to be of unsound mind to commit it. So the puzzle was, if these people were mentally ill, why didn't they go to their doctor? Our National Health Service was, and is, free. I made some enquiries and found that a majority of those who had killed themselves had visited their doctor within three weeks of their death. Obviously, enormously greater numbers had consulted their doctors and not killed themselves, so these three a day could just be the few failures; but it was also possible that at least some of them (plus some of those who hadn't been to their doctor) were not in fact people whose primary need was for medical treatment. But if not medicine or psychiatry, what did they need?

There was only one way to find out for sure: ask them. And there was only one obstacle: no one knew who they were until it was too late.

Lateral thinking suggested to me that though I could not know who *they* were, they could know who *I* was, if I used the media to make everyone in the country aware that I was interested. But interested in what? Satisfying my curiosity? Collecting statistics? People so desperate that they were seriously contemplating taking their own lives could not be treated so frivolously. 'Interested' must mean 'interested to find out if I could help them'.

Assuming that at least some of those whom the cap fitted would learn about my desire to help them and be willing to give it a try, what would they actually do? I would naturally give an address at which they could come and see me or write to me, but in deep distress one wants immediate help and a journey in the middle of the night or from far away might not be easy enough to appeal. It struck me that in an emergency citizens are accustomed to use the telephone. Suicide is undoubtedly an emergency. I studied my telephone. On it was announced EMERGENCY: FIRE POLICE AMBULANCE DIAL 999. Inspiration: what was needed was a sort of 999 for potential suicides, an easily remembered number despairing people could ring at any hour of the day or night. No life-saving service can be part-time to be really effective. One of the weaknesses of the Welfare State was the paucity of people giving other than medical help outside office hours.

Having come to the concept of an emergency service for suicidal people based upon a widely advertised telephone number, but with the offer of a face-to-face visit or correspondence if that was preferred, I began to doubt whether the establishment of it was something I ought to do myself, as I had a more than full time job as Vicar of St Paul Clapham Junction, Chaplain of St John's Hospital Battersea, and Staff Scriptwriter-Visualiser for *Eagle* and *Girl* Magazines, typing scripts until 3 a.m. most nights. If a parson was to make the experiment, it would have to be one with no parishioners, a specialist like most of those in the churches in the City of

London, of which there were three dozen in the square mile around the Bank of England.

While on a busman's holiday at an English Church on the Belgian coast I received an invitation from the Worshipful Company of Grocers to apply for their living of St Stephen Walbrook, Wren's masterpiece next door to the Mansion House.

What would I do there if they appointed me? I told them about my plan for trying to save people from suicide. The successful and intelligent men on the Court asked searching questions and then told me they had decided to appoint me because they thought the experiment worth trying. This was an immense encouragement for years at a time when even I thought I must be mad.

I then went up and down the pubs of Fleet Street telling journalists (many of whom I knew through Marcus Morris and *Eagle*) what a 'human interest' story I had for them, and thanks to them a good start was made towards the achievement by 1984 of 94% of adults knowing about what the *Daily Mirror* decided in 1953 to call a 'Samaritan' service.

Was I the right person?

At this point I realised that if the experiment was at all successful, I would be taking on a lifelong commitment. Why me? Was I a suitable person?

I had one obvious qualification. Logically, it was possible that the three a day who were killing themselves in London might have been helped by counselling – non-medical but still professional. Ever since 1935 I had specialised in counselling on sexual problems, and had become known (not to say notorious) for this. My first job after my ordination in 1935 had been to bury the body of a 14 year old girl who had killed herself when her menstruation started, not knowing what was 'wrong' with her and having no one she could ask. I might have dedicated myself to suicide prevention then and there, providing a network of people you could 'ask' about anything, however embarrassing, but I didn't come to that until later. The vow I made over the grave of that child was, 'Little girl, I never knew you, but you have changed my life. I shall teach kids what I learnt when I was younger than you, even if I get called a dirty old man at the age of 24.' I began that very evening in my parish Youth Club, and I did get called a dirty old man but not by the youngsters. Then, as an unmarried deacon, I began to give talks on sex to young couples about to be married. As word spread, they came from miles around, and when anything went wrong, I was often the one they consulted to put it right. Sexual minorities also began to seek counselling from me.

I not only gained experience of sex therapy but was also often invited to write about human sexuality from a theologically permissive point of view which even now is not invariably found amongst the clergy. One such article the previous year had led to hundreds of people contacting me for help with their sexual problems, and when I came to consider it, I realised that of those of them who had been suicidal, only one needed referral to a psychiatrist. The rest I had been able to help by my counselling. Perhaps I should also be able to help those whose problem was not predominantly sexual.

I had also one obvious *dis*qualification. I was (and am) a cleric, an Anglican priest. Clergy and ministers have acquired for themselves a reputation for being more ready to speak than to listen, for being censorious busybodies, for moralising on subjects they know little about, and for demanding a respect for their opinions and prejudices which they do not accord to those of others. There are many honourable exceptions and I think their number is increasing, but in 1953 if the man in the street was asked who was the *last* person to whom he would Reveal All, outside his own family, he would reply, 'a parson'.

I could only hope that being known as an expert on sexual problems would prevent my clerical collar (which I soon gave up wearing) from being held against me, and that troubled people would feel that they could tell this particular parson anything if thousands of people had found it easy to tell him their most intimate secrets.

In my writings about sex I had never suggested that it doesn't matter what you do. I had maintained that there is only one law, the law of love, and that we all have to try to discover how that one law can best be obeyed by each of us in our own situation which we know better than anyone else. Christians in particular, and liberated human beings in general, are not morally bound by any other rules or prohibitions, though laws may forbid what conscience does not. At that time male homosexuality for example was against the law, which happily no longer criminalises acts between 'consenting adults in private'.

I felt there was a good chance that some suicidal people would come to me if invited, and that a proportion of them would have the kind of problems I knew I could tackle with confidence. The rest could be asked the crucial question with which I began: What sort of help did they need? What kind of attention would be acceptable to them? To what sort of a person did they wish to tell their troubles?

Taking the plunge

For my '999 for the suicidal' I wanted a telephone number to suggest a human emergency for thousands. I knew that the exchange for St Stephen Walbrook would be MANsion House, so I used the telephone (which had been reconnected by the firm repairing the bomb damage) to ask if the number could be changed to MAN 9000. It felt eerie when the operator got me to clean the dial and tell her what number I was speaking from: MAN 9000. We kept it, in addition to the 10 lines on 283 3400, in the form 626 9000, until 1986, when for technical reasons the number of the world's first Hotline for potential suicides had to be abandoned.

I took charge of St Stephen Walbrook on 1 November 1953 having announced that the service for the suicidal would 'soon' start. The first calls came on 2 November, All Souls' Day. I had persuaded my former secretary, Vivien Prosser, to return from Paris to help me. When she arrived and took what she thought was the first call (and describes in *Answers to Suicide*) I had already taken a call from a woman faced with eviction for the nth time who said she was going to kill her four children and then put her head in the gas oven. (One wouldn't now leave emergency telephones unattended: we should despatch our 'flying squad' from his or her home.) I managed to get an extension, but when that ran out I put the mother and boy toddler and elder girl in a cheap hotel, took the younger girl into my home, and drove round in a taxi trying to persuade friends to take the baby, without success, until at last the cabbie stopped at what turned out to be his own house and persuaded his wife to take the baby. Not for the last time the answer was right at hand.

That was really being thrown in at the deep end, but the other calls I took that day only called for a gentle discussion, with more listening than talking.

As the days and weeks went by, it became clear that there were far more callers (up or in) than two of us could cope with, and a growing mailbag as well, not to mention the journalists whom we never put off however busy we were, for without publicity our service would have ground to a halt. Fortunately, the newspaper stories were so appealingly written (even though our strict rule of total confidentiality deprived journalists of fascinating case histories) that in addition to people needing help they attracted people wanting to *give* help. These were of two kinds: professionals, who could be held in reserve, and 'ordinary' people, whom we liked and invited to come regularly, or whom we had doubts about and sent away. Our instinct in this matter was sound but it was some weeks before we discovered what these volunteers could do when given the chance.

The first Samaritans

Those first volunteers, all of whom I still remember vividly, were humble-minded people who did not suppose for a moment that *they* could save lives, but who were kind-hearted enough to want to help *me* and imaginative enough to realise that from what they had read, I must have taken on an impossible job. They saw themselves as being like Lepidus, 'meet to be sent on errands', and were ready to spend hours just giving tea or coffee and an attentive ear to the people who were waiting for the important thing, an interview with me. I am ashamed to say that at that time I fully concurred in their opinion of our relative merits as life-savers, but I've made up for it since.

In fact, it was only a few weeks before I began to suspect that the volunteers, who met every Monday lunchtime for instruction and whom I liked and admired more the more I saw of them, had a much more valuable function than to keep people from getting too impatient and agitated whilst waiting to see me. It was a straightforward matter of observation that the proportion of the callers I actually interviewed diminished, the ones I did see were easier to help because of the time they had spent with a volunteer, and on the whole the people they passed on to me were rightly judged to be in need of a kind of professional attention the volunteers could not give. Eventually I was seeing only about one in eight of those who came, and this proportion was later discovered to be the proportion who, in addition to what we were to call 'befriending', needed counselling or psychotherapy, or referral for psychiatry or other medical treatment.

Of course, human nature being what it is there were some callers who insisted on seeing me and no one else even though they needed only to have someone listen sympathetically to their problems and could just as well have bent the ears of the volunteers – better, in fact, because I was run off my feet and they weren't. But I am glad now that I sometimes had the experience of being with a very distressed person who could have his or her situation transformed not by any of the techniques I was clever at, but by my shutting up and listening with full attention. It was harder for me than for the volunteers, because I *could* do something more impressive and they couldn't, but by being able to manage it with an effort I was the more ready to believe in the value of listening therapy as it slowly became clear that whatever they said, that was what most people really wanted and needed.

It was a great relief to realise that as the service became better known, I would not need to increase my workload to an impossible extent, nor would I need to recruit more than a few other people with similar qualifications to my own. All I would need to do would be to analyse what the best volunteers were doing and select as many more like them as possible and teach them skills which would come naturally to them. I began to eavesdrop whenever I had the opportunity, and also to question Vivien who could be in the same room without making the volunteers self-conscious, as she got on with typing the letters I had dictated whenever there was a moment to spare.

What *did* the volunteers do when they came to take their turn on duty? The answer seemed clear: A great deal of nothing. So what did they *say* when they attached themselves to some tearful or withdrawn or agitated caller? Their most frequent remarks seemed to be: Mmmmmmm. And: How sad. Oh, I *am* sorry. Not to mention: Won't you have another cup of coffee? And, when challenged by the caller: No, not at all – take your time. No, I've nothing else to do – this is what I'm here for. Or, when asked for advice: I wouldn't know what to advise. I'm not any sort of an expert. What do *you* feel would be best?

Their sympathy was human sympathy. I never asked them about their religious beliefs, but I gathered that not all were any kind of believer – not that it mattered, as those that were didn't talk about it. They seemed to know instinctively that any talk of the love of God might be taken as an excuse not to give their own love, and any suggestion of prayer might be regarded as a rebuke if the caller felt deserted by any God there might be. Naturally, this attitude was reinforced by what I said on the subject at our Monday meetings, and by their knowledge that I rejected people who offered to join us if I found them preachy or bossy or prone to give advice or prudish. In those days, my selection was by my own subjective standards and I made some mistakes (it's now objective and sophisticated). My team and I worked on the basis of mutual confidence, and I had looked searchingly into every volunteer's eyes and asked myself the question, If I had done something of which I was horribly ashamed, could I tell it to that face?

Over to the volunteers

I think it was on 2 February 1954 that I called all the volunteers together for a special meeting – certainly it was about three months after starting. 'You miserable so-and-sos,' I said to them, 'how dare you sneak in here when I'm too busy to know what's happening, and start pinching the clients from under my very nose? Nobody asked you to interfere: I had hardly got started on my ministry when you lot came along and started doing the clients more good than I was doing. Only twelve per cent want me, and then only after you've had a go at them: all the rest are foolish enough to prefer *you*. Well, your punishment will be severe. As from now, over to you!

SAMARITAN PRIEST WILL SAVE LIVES said the headline optimistically. Now I know that *you* are the life savers, you are the Samaritans. Never again will I pick up MAN 9000, nor be the one to greet a person who comes to the door. This is now a lay movement for befriending the suicidal and you are the first of what will one day be a worldwide fellowship of Samaritans, meeting a hitherto unrecognised need for someone to *listen.*' They all started talking at once, and I picked out remarks like, 'But what will *you* do? . . . We can't manage without you! . . . We don't know anything about anything! . . . Psychiatrists won't take any notice of us if we try to refer people to them . . .' I was happy to set their fears at rest. I told them that I would still be 'the boss', still choose them, instruct them, discipline them, and if necessary sack them, would still see the people they were unable to help by their befriending alone, and still make all the decisions and all the referrals. In addition, I alone would deal with publicity, and I would still be the one to open the mail. Before long, we settled down into the new pattern. I have taken so much space in recalling these events of more than thirty years ago because they are still relevant. Wherever we exist in the world, we still stand or fall by the befriending, the listening therapy, performed by people who are chosen for their aptitude for that, and for nothing else whatsoever.

What I want to make clear is that The Samaritans are a precise tailor-made answer to a universal need in the lonely, anxious, depressed and suicidal. I did not ask what I wanted to give, but what the clients (as we then called them) wanted to receive. I did ask what I was capable of giving, and discovered that of the two things I could do, the one most in demand was the one that any Samaritan could do, and most could do better than I.

During the next five years, I learnt more about what carefully-selected and well-supervised Samaritans could do, and as their numbers increased I was able to be more and more 'choosy' in turning down any applicants about whom I had any doubts. 'We can't afford to give the benefit of the doubt to anyone who, if they aren't right for the job, may cost a client's life,' was the way I put it, with the full backing of the Samaritans. Indeed, in those years, anyone I accepted was 'on observation' by the tried-and-tested Samaritans before being confirmed as one of us. (They thought it meant they were to observe what went on, and of course they did that too, but the purpose of Observation Duty was so that *we* might observe *them*.)

In addition to becoming more selective about new applicants, I had an occasional purge of existing members. If I found that they were unreliable, unpunctual, or guilty of some fault which could be corrected, I gave them a second chance; but there was no second chance for behaviour which showed that the person wasn't a Samaritan at all. Such things as gossiping about clients' affairs or trying to convert a client to the volunteer's religion or philosophy or arranging secret meetings with a client outside the centre led to instant dismissal. This did not of course take anyone by surprise: on being accepted, the Samaritan was given a document to sign promising *i.a.* obedience to instructions and total confidentiality of anything communicated by a client from everyone outside the organisation. The document also contained the words, 'I understand that my membership may be terminated at any time without notice or reason given by myself or by the Director.' People normally knew the reasons, but by the agreement that they would not be stated, much fruitless argument was avoided. As we have grown, and times have changed, and the relationship between the Director and the volunteers is unlikely to be that of guru and disciples, reasons for dismissal may now sometimes be given, and as far as I know no one has sued for defamation.

I do not consider that every Director should necessarily be the kind of 'benevolent dictator' that I was for 21 years in the London (now Central London) Branch, but I do hold that procedures worked out over the years in accordance with the conclusion after full discussion 'The needs of the client dictate that we do so-and-so,' ought not to be abandoned without very good reason. Anyone who carelessly makes changes for the sake of change or to show contempt for the accumulated wisdom of the movement, is unworthy to be in a position to do this, like a vandal defacing a noble edifice with his undistinguished name or vulgar slogans. For instance, in the first few weeks I started a tradition, which I hoped would be continued for ever, of giving each Samaritan an individual number which would not only replace his or her surname for the sake of anonymity, but would also distinguish one John or Susan from another John or Susan, be a useful record of seniority in the Branch, and enable every Samaritan throughout the world to be known by his or her unique personal number within the Branch plus the number of the Branch in the country plus the number of the country. (It is on this basis that I am known as 'Chad 1/1/1'.) I feel sure it was people neither knowing nor caring what traditions I had established, rather than a malicious desire to frustrate my hopes, which caused certain Branches to abandon these unique numbers and instead refer to John 1, John 2, John 3, Susan 1, Susan 2, Susan 3 . . . it only requires a few Branches to do this for the whole tradition to be destroyed. I hope that even now they will heed my appeal to return to the original concept.

Samaritans, being hand-picked for their niceness, are seldom power-seekers. They sometimes have a rather selfish desire to avoid boring administrative tasks and confine themselves to the heart-warming or heart-rending work with the callers. We have to tell them that it is for the sake of the *callers* that administration has to be done efficiently. In the early days we elected to the Committee the most exemplary Samaritans we could find, overruling their protests, and never gave power to people who seemed to want it.

Beginning to spread

From 1959, other centres of Samaritan work were set up, the late Revd Professor James Blackie being responsible for taking the initiative in the northern capital, Edinburgh, and the late Christopher Pepys (subsequently Bishop of Buckingham) in Liverpool. Glasgow and Aberdeen quickly followed in Scotland, and Manchester (rescued after a shaky start by the late Revd Basil Higginson) in England; and in the same year, 1960, we became international. Mr Andrew Tu had set up a service in Hong Kong in 1958 which adopted our methods and joined us in 1960, when Mr Nadir Dinshaw of the London Branch inspired the creation of Branches in Karachi (now, alas, no longer functioning) and Bombay (still going strong), whilst

Dean (now Canon) Gonville ffrench-Beytagh began a Branch in what was then Salisbury Rhodesia and is now Harare Zimbabwe. All these centres were in touch with me and committed themselves firmly to the Samaritan name and such Samaritan principles as giving primacy to Befriending by selected volunteers supervised by someone with professional qualifications of some sort, the volunteers being chosen without regard to religion, class, politics or race and being forbidden to try to convert the callers to their own views.

It may surprise some readers to know that although the telephone was a most convenient method of effortless (and, if desired, anonymous) approach to us in developed countries, it was recognised even then that what made a centre 'Samaritan' was not the use of an emergency telephone, but the nature of the person chosen to encounter the client whether he or she rang up, or came in(with or without appointment), or asked us to pay him a visit, or wrote to us. If the person responding to a cry for help was a volunteer selected for suitability for our befriending therapy, then the centre could be recognised as Samaritan; and if not, not.

By April 1963 there were another 14 centres, all of them in touch with me (and, as it happens, all in the United Kingdom and therefore making much use of their emergency telephone numbers, which even then were specially allocated by the Post Office, e.g. CALedonian 3333 for Edinburgh and BLAckfriars 9000 for Manchester.) All the then recognised centres, including the four in other countries, banded together into a Company Limited by Guarantee permitted to omit the word 'Limited' (hence The Samaritans *Inc.*) which was registered with the Charity Commissioners as a Charity. I was elected Chairman, and although all the representatives of the UK Branches (obviously the Asian and African ones could not often attend meetings) respected my original initiative and above all my discovery of Befriending, the fact that they had developed without my constant guidance for up to four years meant that they had in some cases evolved certain idiosyncratic ways which they tended to cherish. I was anxious that we should start as we meant to go on, and offer the same service everywhere, so that there were sometimes clashes when deciding what practices were optional and what were essential. (No Branch now questions the 7 Principles and 7 Practices adapted from the various versions of The Twenty Principles.)

At about the same time, unknown to us for another couple of years, a nineteen-year-old engineer called Jacques André Conchon set up an emergency befriending service for the suicidal in São Paulo, Brazil, called at first Companha, and later Centro, da Valorização da Vida (Company, or Centre, for the validification of life). When he and I met, we realised that our ideas were the same, and I had the privilege of travelling all over Brazil and South America, often with Jacques Conchon, from the time he had three Branches to the time he had over 60, teaching the principles of befriending. Eventually 'CVV' changed its name to 'CVV-Samaritanos', and Brazil is the biggest country (in terms of the number of Branches) in Befrienders International, and second only to the British Isles in the whole Samaritan movement. The sad thing is that Latin America has not so far produced a leader of the calibre of Jacques Conchon.

It may be imagined that in 1963 I had my hands full with the work of Director of what has always been the biggest Branch, at the time of its fastest growth by doubling up each year, plus the work of being the movement's spokesman in the media, plus trying to guide the Branches (themselves rapidly increasing in number) as Chairman. But it was an immensely stimulating time, and I was thrilled to be in a position to communicate the vision I had had and the discovery I had made in the early months and refined and proved effective ever since, with the authority of elected Chairman as well as the moral authority of 'the Founder'. During the next three years, although occasionally depressed by the ambivalence shown towards me by some colleagues, I was on the whole exhilarated by our success and our generous acceptance by the medical and other professionals, and looked forward to reaping the reward of the early struggles, when I was always overworked and having to manage on a shoestring, by being able to delegate to trusted lieutenants and to have the wherewithal to pay for the burden to be eased. But these and other hopes were dashed.

A rash decision

At the meeting at which I was re-elected Chairman by 20 votes to 4, our Consultant Psychiatrist, Dr Richard Fox, told me he was worried by the amount of negative ambivalence I had to bear, and when I said that my shoulders were broad, he suggested that a change of Chairman might unite the movement. I took a lot of notice of him because he had stuck his neck out to praise our lay volunteers and their befriending therapy and to defend to his psychiatric colleagues our close involvement as non-medical non-professionals with the suicidal. He had greatly helped me in my efforts to give the Samaritans confidence in the value and efficacy of what they were doing, provided they had good supervision and back-up, and when you are put on some sort of a pedestal there are few people to whom you can talk as man to man. (It is still true that I am the only person who can never ring The Samaritans however distressed I might be.) I was touched by his concern for me and for the movement, and the following year, with still only four people preferring a change, I announced that I would not stand for election again. One who had *not* desired a change, the late Revd Dr 'Bill' Thomson of Belfast, whom I had got to know well when I had said they should not start until all denominations were ready to work together as leaders, was elected Chairman. (His colleague from 1961 and his successor, the Revd Sidney Callaghan, was deservedly awarded the OBE in 1984.)

I suspect that my decision to stand down would have been different if I had known beforehand that I was not to be a member of the Executive Committee. I was made a Permanent Member of the Council of Management, but felt that, for all practical purposes, the movement I had created was thenceforward to be shaped by other minds than mine. When the organisation began to prosper I would sometimes remember the days when it ran only on my personal overdraft, and when a taxi fare to meet a client could mean my not being able to afford any lunch the next day. It is no disparagement of dear good 'Bill' or of his successors as Chairman to say that to a great extent the movement was cut off from its original inspiration; and that well as it has done, it might have done even better if I had been allowed to participate in the discussions of the Executive, where I could easily have been outvoted if I became tiresome.

Almost my last participation in an Executive decision was in 1967, when I was outvoted on a matter I felt was of vital inportance to the welfare of the clients and to our unimpeded spread throughout the world.

Rival concepts on the Continent

In the autumn of 1960 I travelled to Vienna in the roundabout way which became typical of my journeys. I first visited Mrs Nuran Ulupinar in Istanbul to see if her voluntary psychiatric clinics ought to be taken under the wing of The Samaritans. Before this could happen she remarried and emigrated to England. Then I went to Athens to ask Archbishop Damascinos' help in starting a Branch there. The contacts he gave me never did get going. Then via Rome, where we didn't at that time have a Branch, to Geneva for the train to Nyon and a Conference at Château de Bossey, organised by the Swiss crisis line La Main Tenduë and paid for by a Paris business man, M. Georges Lillaz. I arrived in the middle of the opening address in French, English and German by the late Revd Ernst Schwyn, who interrupted himself to call out, 'Welcome to our beloved Founder, Chad Varah!' The representatives of Switzerland, Germany, France, Belgium and Holland, and the five other Samaritans including David Arthur, stood and cheered. I gulped, and muttered thanks, and refrained from saying, 'I did *not* found the organisations represented here which ignore the principles of The Samaritans.' I more often regret being insincerely polite than being honestly rude. We seemed to disagree about everything: with the nice French Protestant who ran SOS L'Amitié par Téléphone in Paris about working only with paid professionals from a secret address; with Die Dargebotene Hand which in Zürich had an enormous switchboard enabling devoted Salvation Army people to transfer all calls to one of thirty experts in their offices; and most of all with Telefonseelsorge (pastoral care by telephone) which was explicitly a Diakonische Werk (deaconing work) of the German Churches.

We failed to convince the other organisations of the importance of befriending, or even to get some of their representatives to grasp what it was – a particular form of therapy, and not the face-to-face work of which they seemed so afraid. The Germans denied any evangelistic intent but would only enlist devout Churchfolk; I guess some really did avoid preaching, but others were blissfully unaware when they were doing it.

We agreed to join a Centre International d'Information des Services de Secours d'Urgence par Téléphone, with Protestant Pastor Raynauld Martin of Geneva as Secretary, as we did not see what harm could be done by exchange of information – it might even lead to some of our Continental friends learning the marvels of Befriending and wishing to join our movement. How could we have known that the result would be that Befriending would be kept out of Continental Europe and that after a quarter of a century we should still have only a handful of Branches there?

The second gathering of the Centre International d'Information was in 1962 at Bad Boll theological seminary near Stuttgart, with the Revd Otto Kehr of Telefonseelsorge as President. Samaritan delegates felt like fish out of water. The charts on the wall showed that with Telefonseelsorge the commonest problem was 'spiritual problems' and bottom of the list was 'depression'. The Samaritan chart naturally showed the exact opposite.

In 1964 it was England's turn to have the Conference and mine (as Chairman of The Samaritans, incorporated the previous year) to be President. We met at Christ Church Oxford and found that Samaritans had hardly anything in common with the continental delegates – except for the Samaritan-minded Dr Martonová from Czechoslovakia, whom Richard Fox and I were later to visit in Prague.

For the next three years it was my duty to preside over the meetings of the International Committee of the 'Centre d'Information' at Waterloo in Belgium, where I was almost always in a minority of one; because I *knew* what the clients wanted if they were to be saved from suicide, and the others knew what the Church could offer (and in Sweden that meant priests only) and what the clients therefore needed and 'ought to want' (though it was seldom put so crudely). Looking back now, I can see what a threat I must have seemed to be to these mostly good if blinkered men to whom it was obvious that a humane unbeliever could not possibly be compared with a professing Christian, however uncaring; and who in many cases depended on running a Church-based service if the Church was to pay the costs and their salaries. (My own salary came from my Church work, and still does; neither I nor anyone else was paid to do Samaritan work. The Church of England has been very tolerant about the time I have devoted to a purely humanitarian cause.)

There was only one thing I and the rest of the International Committee could have rightly said to one another, and that was 'Good-bye.' Unfortunately, in 1967 in Brussels, when the Revd Fr Rémi Mens took over from me as President, we said just the opposite – instead of a simple information centre we would become a Federation, with the voting rigged so that The Samaritans, whose Branches by then outnumbered all the rest put together, would always have a minority of the votes. Instead of Samaritan Befriending spreading through Europe, The Samaritans would be prohibited from setting up Branches in the territory of members of the 'International Federation of Telephone Emergency Services' (IFOTES).

I told my Samaritan colleagues we should have nothing to do with it. They disagreed. 'Let us continue the dialogue,' they said. I was no longer Chairman, and was outvoted. I had had three years of failure of dialogue. I hadn't been allowed to discuss with the ordinary volunteers on the Continent, some of whom must have been unofficial Samaritans. I hadn't even been allowed to communicate with the *Branches* of Telefonseelsorge etc. to find out what they actually did for the clients – the national organisation forbade their members to reply to the President. This was a shrewd precaution because, on the rare occasions when I have been invited to an IFOTES centre (e.g. Amsterdam, Antwerp, Dortmund, Münster, Hagen, Lübeck, Turin, Venice, Genoa, Montpellier, Nice, Clermont-Ferrand), many of the volunteers have seemed to me to think along Samaritan lines, and showed no signs of the hostility displayed by official delegates.

The Samaritans tried. Oh, how they tried! And for how long: seventeen years. They gave their best people to be on the International Committee: the Revd John Eldrid (my assistant in the early days and again in preparation for taking over from me as Director of the London Branch in 1974; twice Chairman of The Samaritans Inc.; Vice-President of IFOTES) and Jean Burt, MBE (an even older member of the London Branch than John, now retired from being General Secretary of The Samaritans), who became Treasurer of IFOTES. Both are outstanding Samaritans and much more tactful than I, but even they could not and did not change the implacable opposition to our mission to spread our Samaritan Befriending to every place in the world where suicide is a problem.

The IASP

I mentioned that the journey in 1960 from Istanbul which took me to Geneva for a conference of continental Church-based services was to bring me home by way of Vienna. Here, a far-sighted clergyman, Prälat Leopold Ungar, in charge of a Roman Catholic welfare organisation called Caritas, had asked the Professor of Psychiatry, Dr Erwin Ringel, to set up a clinic for suicidal people in the late 40s. By 1960, Dr Ringel and his colleagues had acquired a great deal of knowledge of the pre-suicidal state, but knew that much more research was needed, so a conference was called in the University Clinic in Spitalgasse to which I was invited, seven years after my pioneering a hotline for the suicidal. All the other participants were psychiatrists or psychologists, but I was glad to be there to make sure that one paper was concerned with giving practical help to despairing persons who were not straightforward psychiatric cases. The only Samaritan with me was Mrs Ulupinar, who spoke excellent English but, as the proceedings were in German, could make no contribution. Dr Ringel later learnt to speak English fluently, but it took longer for him to learn to value the contribution of volunteers, and to stop concluding every discussion of Befriending with the pronouncement, 'Alles muss aber ärtzlich getan worden' (but everything must be done medically).

The Vienna Congress led to the foundation of the International Association for Suicide Prevention, which grew steadily until some of its biennial congresses attracted a thousand delegates. Dr Richard Fox joined in 1964 as an individual member and The Samaritans as corporate members, on the strength of which Dr Fox became Vice-President of IASP before his retirement from Samaritan work. Congresses of IASP have been held in Copenhagen, Basel, Los Angeles, London, Amsterdam, Jerusalem, Helsinki, Paris, Caracas and Vienna again for the 25th anniversary. At all of these except Copenhagen, I and other Samaritans presented papers (except that in Caracas Nat Smith, Chairman of The Samaritans Inc., took my place). The only ones at which I spoke at a Plenary Session were Los Angeles in 1967 and London in 1969. I was told that my lecture on the use of volunteers in Los Angeles began the transformation of much of the work in the United States, which had been either psychiatric or Church-based with unselected volunteers, so that there gradually emerged professional services which made great use of volunteers selected by Samaritan methods to such essentially Samaritan befriending work. The famous Suicide Prevention Center of Los Angeles, which will forever be associated with the work of Dr Edwin Shneidman, Dr Farberow and Dr Robert Litman, began operations with a dozen psychiatrists holding a DPM and a dozen psychologists with PhDs, but after a few years entrusted most of the crisis work in the first instance to 'clinical associates' whom I found it impossible to distinguish from Samaritans. A similar spirit is found in San Francisco, where the Professor of Psychiatry, Dr Jerome Motto, is living proof that one can be an outstanding professional and a true Samaritan, and in many other places where the American Association of Suicidology (which honoured me with their Louis I. Dublin Award in 1974) as the US section of IASP maintains a high standard in all its affiliated Branches. Special mention must be made of San Mateo and of Charlotte Ross, outstanding trainer of volunteers and a leading light of IASP. It must be said that although IASP started in Europe it is the Americans who have been its great strength, and few of the countries in which it has national associations can compare these with the AAS. Indeed, there are few centres outside the USA where IASP maintains hotlines, and the contribution of IASP to suicide prevention continues to be chiefly through research. I should like to see this begin to change. The research we need in order to be able to help people effectively has been done, and I think we should get on with it. Perhaps the

Congress in San Francisco in 1987 will, submerged in ever more and more recondite statistics, experience a widespread demand for a plan of *action* to combat suicide throughout the world.

Rival concepts in the Antipodes

It wasn't only in Europe that those who apparently believed that Christ had made the wrong person the hero of the Parable of the Good Samaritan set up rival organisations. In Sydney, Australia, the Revd Ted Noffs (later of the Wayside Chapel, Kings Cross, Sydney) had heard about The Samaritans, and told me that in 1962 he had pressed the Revd Alan Walker, Minister of the Central Methodist Mission to start a Branch, but that this Minister, a forceful preacher who was subsequently knighted, had decided to re-invent the whole thing as 'a Christian movement: it would only accept people who confessed Jesus Christ as Saviour and Lord'. It would be called 'Life Line' and the volunteers would be chosen from committed Christians who would pledge themselves to seek every opportunity to bring the client to Jesus Christ – the very thing which would disqualify a person from being accepted as a Samaritan. In the book *Life Line* the birth of the idea is given as a suicidal call on a Saturday from one Roy who was invited to come and hear the Minister preach the next day and did so, and on the Tuesday gassed himself leaving a note saying he was 'leaving the world unwanted, unloved and without hope'. One can sympathise deeply with the Minister's failure – we have all had failures – while still wondering how, after Roy had written to him 'a job and £150 would have saved me,' he could still begin the Life Line Manual with the words 'The supreme purpose of the Life Line Centre is to lead men and women to Christ.' Samaritans believe that this purpose is likely to drive some callers to suicide.

Fortunately, not all the places to which Life Line spread through the Methodist network in eastern Australia (we have The Samaritans in the west) adopted the sock-it-to-them approach. Indeed, one centre was criticised for accepting Jewish members and another for not enquiring whether applicants were agnostic, and several that I visited were more like Samaritan Branches than like Sydney, but would never break with Sydney. The irrational loyalty to an organisation whose ideas one rejects has been studied by psychologists. In the case of cults, deprogramming has sometimes been effective. To some extent, 'continuing the dialogue' has been possible in Australia and South Africa, because contact was not with the international leadership, which continues to be hardline Christian, but with individual Branches and their members, some of whom, like many in Europe, have learnt from the best teachers of all – the callers. What can one say, though, about a certain crisis line in Taiwan consisting almost entirely of Buddhists and agnostics, which was affiliated to an evangelistic Christian organisation, without its knowledge let alone its consent, by a missionary just before his leaving the country, but which, when informed of this, decided to continue the affiliation?

The early Sixties were a bad time from the point of view of the setting up of 'suicide prevention and crisis intervention centres' based on a religious perversion of pure Samaritan doctrine. And it was easy for them to spread through a ready-made network of Churches with people, premises and money, whereas we always had to create an humanitarian service from scratch. By 1986 the number of non-Samaritan and anti-Samaritan centres in the world was at least double that of the Samaritan Branches, though some of the former were ephemeral and very few of ours fell by the wayside. No country showed a dramatic reduction in the suicide rate except the UK and a few other places where we had been working long and intensively enough to make an impact. If a country of twenty million people has a suicide rate of 15 per 100,000 per annum, i.e. 3,000 persons, and a parasuicide rate of ten times as many, i.e. another 30,000 persons, it is idle to hope for a measurable reduction of the suicide rate if you are attending only a couple of thousand clients a year of whom only 5 per cent are suicide risks.

Our philosophy

The reader will by now be aware that Befriending, this listening therapy discovered, developed, refined and practised by The Samaritans, is not merely a method of making those receiving it less likely to kill themselves, but also a philosophy and a way of life. Some volunteers have gone so far as to say that 'Samaritanism' is their religion, but it isn't necessary to go so far in order to be deeply influenced by the concept in one's living away from our Centres.

The Samaritan philosophy, which is in fact the flowering of my own personal philosophy, is based on respect and tolerance for others. This is easier for the born Samaritans, who have a natural humility that leads them to consider themselves no more important (though of course no less) than the human being they are privileged to try to help.

The caller is often a person who does not even receive attention from his fellows, let alone respect. When he encounters a Samaritan, he soon realises, often with incredulity, that this kindly stranger is interested in him and is willing to listen to his troubles. At first he will often pause to give the opportunity which even the nicest people 'outside' seem to demand, for the other to chip in with experiences of his or her own. Encountering only an enquiring expression or a gentle question, he confides a little more; and eventually, if all goes well, the whole story pours out in a way it probably never has before. This is in itself therapeutic. (Our previously neglected caller must not be confused with the person avid for attention who announces impressively that she is going to confide something which she has never told anyone else, which might be flattering if you didn't suspect she's told *every*one else.)

The Samaritan has not only been listening, but has also been conveying respect for the caller's right to be the person he is, and tolerance of those things in him which are in contrast to the character and opinions and behaviour of the Samaritan. The greater the difference between two human beings whose attitude proclaims '*vive la différence*', the more obvious it is that the one cannot *advise* the other. 'If I were you, I should do so-and-so' is in any case nonsense, because if I were you I would obviously do whatever you in fact did; and if it means 'If I were in your position . . .' then it is irrelevant, because you might want to do something which the caller would find unappealing, or beyond his power, or wrong.

Professional counsellors turn any request for advice with the question 'What do *you* think you should do?' because they are as convinced that the client should face issues and make decisions as a teacher is that a child should do its own sums. The motivation of the Samaritan is less didactic: he honestly does not feel qualified to guide the caller, any more than to sit in judgment on him.

Patience is what is required to allow a child to read or walk, or a person who has had a stroke or has a speech defect to express himself, or to allow a suspicious or disturbed person to come round to the idea of trusting us, or to permit a person embarrassed about what he needs to tell someone to take a little time to decide that we shall not despise or ridicule him. You do not 'insult' anyone by being patient with him: you are not treating him as a child or as a mentally incompetent person, but as a human being who needs help, and has indicated this by getting in touch with The Samaritans.

The word 'patience' is derived from the Latin word for suffering, and those who would befriend the suicidal are in fact those who are willing to suffer, and suffer with, fellow human beings in distress. Only people who are acting the part of Lady Bountiful, admiring herself doing good works, pretend that they are never bored or exasperated or even tempted to be resentful of the self-centredness which unhappiness often produces in the callers. Anyone who never finds befriending an effort just hasn't been paying attention or lacks imagination.

It is sometimes said that the old are too patient in the sense of uncomplaining, and that the young have a divine impatience which urges them to put all the ills of the world right, by yesterday. This is obviously true in some cases, but the difference is not really one of age, rather it is of the wisdom which age is supposed to bring but doesn't always, and which the young are supposed not yet to have attained but which in our day they surprisingly often display. Like everyone else, those of the young who are not apathetic are divided into the impatient, who are eager for action and tend to be attracted to ideologies and revolutionary or religious panaceas, and the patient, who remain in touch with reality, allow themselves to think and feel, and do something of practical help to some actual persons. Many of the latter join The Samaritans, whose philosophy appeals to them and who have not had their tolerance destroyed by being set in their ways. Any country ought to be proud of its young Samaritans.

Between the fanatics who have the answers for everyone else, and the Samaritans who want to help people to find their own answers, there is such a great gulf fixed that any attempt to co-operate would be a waste of time. Those who 'know' that 'Jesus is the answer' (whatever this may mean) before they have heard the question, seem to Samaritans to be terribly insecure people using slogans to avoid facing the complexity of human existence; and doubtless they in their turn see Samaritan tolerance as indifference to sin, and Samaritan recognition of the goodness in all sorts and conditions of men to be apostasy. Between those two attitudes there is no fence to sit on and no compromise possible: the sharper the conflict, the clearer the issues, the more chance people have of choosing the side that really suits their character and outlook.

The second decade

All this time that people seeking to serve their prejudices were playing politics, the good thing was that the idea was steadily spreading that if you were so unhappy you were thinking you might kill yourself, there was no sense or merit in suffering in silence – you should unburden yourself to someone, and if your own family and circle of friends wouldn't do or didn't seem to want to know, or if you *had* no family or friends, then you had a standing invitation to turn to The Samaritans (or, in the countries where we were not yet operating, to some crisis intervention service which might well have some Samaritan types working for it whether they were chosen for this or were likely to be dismissed if it was discovered). I was happy that by the mid-sixties, about the time that I edited the first book in the series of which this is the latest, it had become more and more widely accepted that there was no shame in seeking help, that the 'stiff upper lip' was psychologically inadvisable except in peril, and most important of all, that the person you turned to did not need to be someone with qualifications or diplomas so long as he or she *cared*. People began to talk about 'the caring professions', too, so that in principle if the enthusiastic amateur was out of his depth and persuaded you to go to a doctor or other professional, you would still be with a caring person. I'm not sure at what date the noun 'carer' began to be used, and it's a bit awkward, but it was good that the term 'uncaring' should have become such a pejorative expression and those who rule us be constantly reminded that *little* brother was watching them for signs of this.

Samaritans had used their influence behind the scenes to get the law which made suicide a felony changed, in 1961. Much of the credit should go to our late beloved Presidents, Dr Doris Odlum, who died in 1986, and to her predecessor, Professor Erwin Stengel (in whose memory the IASP gives an annual prize). It was obvious that if there was *any* chance that someone who survived a suicidal act might be prosecuted and imprisoned (even though in the rare cases where the police prosecuted, the usual result was the granting of probation on condition that the person agreed to enter a mental hospital as a voluntary patient), people thinking of suicide would be nervous about admitting this.

The Samaritans do not seek to be 'a power in the land' but to serve individuals humbly and secretly. They rarely feel able to press for a change in the law, and then only when it is clear that without a change people will be driven to suicide. Two laws desired by Samaritans, whatever their personal beliefs or predilections, because they were 'what the needs of the clients dictate', were the Abortion Act of 1967 and the Act which implemented those recommendations of the Wolfenden Committee (backed up by the Church of England Moral Welfare Council as well as by The Samaritans) making male homosexual acts 'by consenting adults in private' no longer criminal (as, thanks to Queen Victoria's blissful ignorance, female homosexual acts had never been).

We all knew of girls and women who had killed themselves because they could not obtain an abortion properly performed, or who had died at the hands of an unqualified operator, so whatever the private beliefs of some Samaritans, all of them were 'pro-choice' for the clients. Our RC volunteers especially would have liked the way Rosalynn Carter put it in her *First Lady from Plains* in 1984: 'Jimmy was more conservative about the abortion issue. I oppose it for myself, but I have a hard time with deciding for other women what is right or wrong or best for them.' A few fanatical anti-abortionists infiltrated our ranks, as did a few anti-sex campaigners for censorship of adults' reading and viewing, but they soon exposed themselves by accusing their colleagues of 'persuading girls to murder their unborn children' or by suggesting that female volunteers who tried to deal constructively with sex-callers were either prostitutes or doing it for kicks. Needless to say, Samaritans are chosen because they are not the type of people whose nature is to try to impose their own beliefs on distressed callers, so they would neither recommend nor condemn abortion, but would only include it among the options open to a caller with an unwanted pregnancy. It always causes painful embarrassment if someone gets up at one of our schools or conferences and proclaims something totally un-Samaritan: Samaritans are the nicest people you will ever meet, but threaten the interests of the clients and they are rightly capable of enquiring of the offender's colleagues, 'You don't have *selection* of volunteers in your Branch, then?'

We had all encountered male callers who were suicidal because they could not accept their homosexuality or had been shamed by being exposed to their families or colleagues at a time when 'coming out' was unheard of, or were being blackmailed by some heartless avaricious character who had discovered their 'guilty' secret, so even those of our volunteers who *at that time* could be excused for ignorance of the facts about homosexuality and found prejudices within themselves were unable to maintain their disapproval when actually befriending someone who turned out not to be any kind of monster but just another human being. From the beginning I had made it clear that homosexuality was no bar to being accepted as a Samaritan volunteer, if suitable. Like so many Samaritan attitudes, it might be taken for granted now but required moral courage then.

Getting together

Exchange of experiences between volunteers, as distinct from their representatives who met at Council Meetings after 1963, was facilitated by our holding annual conferences. The first, in 1961, was at Balliol College Oxford, the second at St Mary's College Durham, and the third (the first one after we became a Company) at Sheffield, where Dr Stengel was Professor of

Psychiatry. The fourth was at Christ Church Oxford and was a little overshadowed by the international gathering I have already described, and reduced in numbers by our hiving off the north for an alternative conference in Dundee. In 1965 we returned to the one conference for the whole movement, at Manchester University. At the conference in Cardiff in 1966, Bill Thomson took over from me as Chairman. Subsequent annual conferences under a succession of Chairmen were held in Glasgow, Southampton, Keele, Exeter, Leeds, Stirling, York, Manchester again, Lancaster, Loughborough, and from 1977 always at York. Loughborough stands out in my memory because it was the only conference after relinquishing the chair at which I have ever been invited to speak at a plenary, and York in 1973 because Sir Keith Joseph opened it and over coffee was kind enough to say to me that one of his staff had told him we saved the Government about two millions a year by keeping people out of hospital and/or fit to work. 'No, no,' I said quickly, 'we cannot accept your generous offer of two millions a year because it's much more than we need. But if I may introduce you to our Bursar, he'll tell you what much more modest amount we *do* need . . .' That was the beginning of our Government grant, which we took as official approval of our activities, and used for enabling Samaritans to attend conferences and 'schools', as we wanted the Branches to be self-supporting *and* to pay a levy to cover necessary administration.

Our 'Schools for Leaders' proved so valuable that in 1972 they were duplicated, being held that year at Swanwick and at the University of East Anglia, and from 1977 triplicated, but always at Swanwick. Lately there has been a School in two parts for Publicity Officers and for Fund Raisers.

The increasing number of Branches had necessitated division into a dozen Regions whose representatives formed the Executive just as the representatives of the Branches formed the Council of Management. Each Region tended to have a conference at least once a year with a very large attendance in some cases. The extension of our work from the UK into the Republic of Ireland (whose first Branch, Dublin, was no. 110) allowed one of these Regions to be simply 'Ireland', for the things which separate the north and the south no more separate Samaritans than do the conflicts in the north, where no caller has ever asked about the religious or political persuasion of the Samaritan who answers, and where it has become standard procedure for bomb-warnings to be communicated to the police through The Samaritans. Scotland is another Region, and like Ireland has 15 Branches. England and Wales are divided into North (9 Branches), North East (16), North West (15), East Midlands (10), Midlands & North Wales (15), South Wales and the Marches (10), East (15), London (15), South East (15), South (16), South West (10).

Administration has always been kept to a miminum, and is done very efficiently and economically from a converted house in Slough, where the Revd David Evans succeeded the late Revd Basil Higginson and on the retirement of Miss Jean Burt, MBE, as Joint General Secretary, Simon Armson was appointed in 1984 to assist him.

It is difficult to keep this account strictly chronological as it is easier to follow if we sometimes mention later developments, but all we need note to complete the period up to the formation of The Samaritans Inc. in 1963 is that the founding Branches were Aberdeen, Belfast, Bombay, Bournemouth, Brighton (discontinued, and later re-started), Cambridge, Dundee, Edinburgh, Glasgow, Hull, Jersey, Karachi (discontinued), Kowloon Hong Kong (expelled, replaced by Wanchai Hong Kong), Liverpool, London, Manchester, Portsmouth, Reading, Salisbury Rhodesia, Stoke on Trent and Woolwich (discontinued). There were at that time also 16 Probationary Branches and 15 Preparatory Groups.

Those who have held the position of Chairman have been, since I resigned, Bill Thomson 1966–8, John Eldrid 1968–72, David Arthur 1972–6, Michael Yorke 1976–9, Nancy Kerr 1979–82, Nat Smith 1982–5 and Albert Jewell, 1985–.

Important developments

All we need note to complete the period between the formation of The Samaritans Inc. and the separation from it of our Branches outside the British Isles to form a sister organisation in 1974 called Befrienders International (The Samaritans Worldwide) are three outstanding developments, one at the beginning and two at the end of the period.

At the time of the formation of the Company, the London Branch, by now very busy and having a small staff paid for by a grant from the Calouste Gulbenkian Foundation, was still operating very inconveniently from the outer and inner vestries of the Church and from rooms up the tower to which led what people call a spiral staircase though of course it's helical. On the first floor, Night Watch slept; on the second, John Eldrid and our Psychiatric Social Worker Mary Bruce had their offices; and on the third, up 55 steps, my secretary and I had our offices. In 1963 someone gave some new (well, less threadbare) linoleum for what had been my study (and now is again). Taking up the old stuff, I found a trap door which, when opened, showed a sort of well or pit about eight feet deep with mud at the bottom. I lowered myself gingerly into the well, and found from near the bottom of it a tunnel about eighteen inches high running eastwards. I crawled with difficulty along it and was soon in complete blackness and could recognise human bones and decayed coffin wood only by the feel. Eventually I came to a point where my hands went over an edge into a void, and when I shouted at it, I got an echo which indicated that this was quite an extensive vault. As I did not care to dive head first into it, I went back to the original pit and turned round and re-entered the tunnel backwards, so that I could hang over the edge at the end by my hands. When I did this, my feet were not touching the floor, and I thought it prudent to scramble up again and come back with someone else and a rope. However, it proved not to be possible to scramble back, so hoping there was not a well 200 feet deep below me, which even without crocodiles would have been alarming, I let go – and fell about four inches. Then I flicked on my cigarette lighter (it was a few years before I gave up smoking) and found myself in an almost disused burial vault. There were three or four mouldering coffins near me, and I managed to pile one on top of another to climb back to civilisation. It was this space, which unfortunately extended only under the vestries and the very west end of the church, which was imaginatively converted by Donald Armstrong Smith, at the cost of the Worshipful Company of Grocers, to make most attractive premises for the Branch, still named 'Grocers' Gift'.

No matter what it said over the entrance, the Samaritans persisted in referring to 'the Crypt', reserving the name 'Grocers' Gift' for the wide, arched, whitewashed area in the middle which was supposed to be called the common room. It was a lovely place, with a peaceful, perhaps womb-like feel about it, and was not only elegant but cosy, with 'Ern' (the urn) bubbling and hissing. Other Branches have reminiscences too, but I felt my own, of the founding Branch, would be of general interest. It was unfortunately necessary to divide this space in the late seventies into a utility room and three additional Befriending Rooms named for George (Millington, Chairman of the Branch for the first 12 years that it had one), the late Godfrey (Gooch, whose legacy allowed us to purchase our West End Annexe at 3 Hornton Place, Kensington), and the late Diana (Churchill, a full-time unpaid worker until her tragic death).

The Central London Branch is now seeking premises big enough to replace both the Crypt and Hornton Place.

'The Befrienders'

Grocers' Gift was the scene of the other important event, towards the end of that decade. In 1971 I had a visit from the late Harry W. Junkin, a Canadian television writer who had made his name and fortune by scripting 'The Saint' for television. Now he wished to do something serious and altruistic, and was attracted to The Samaritans. He was totally captivated by the spirit of Grocers' Gift and by the volunteers, and invented two female and two male volunteers to feature in each of a series of stories to be called 'The Befrienders'. All he needed now was the case histories which he proposed to extract from us. He was nonplussed when I told him all our information about callers was confidential, and was on the point of abandoning the idea when I said, 'My dear fellow, *you* are a creative writer. All you have to do is to create characters and situations for them to be in, and if I consider these suicidal, bowl them at me and I will answer in a Samaritan way into your tape recorder.' 'OK,' he said, 'if a man had an invalid wife whom he loved, but because of her disability he also had a mistress, and this mistress suddenly insisted that he put his wife into a home and have her to live with him openly, could he become suicidal?' 'Yes,' I replied. 'Right,' said Harry, 'I am that man, and you are a Samaritan called . . . er . . . Janet.' Then he switched on his tape.

Janet was played by Megs Jenkins, and the other 'Samaritans' by Michael Culver, Peter Armstrong and Jane Wellow. Many famous actors took part in the eleven episodes: I remember especially Gordon Jackson as a police officer trying in vain to get information about a murderer from Janet, and in episode no. 6, which I scripted myself ('Nobody Understands Miranda') Jean Marsh played excellently the girl who thought she was depressed because she'd lost her boyfriend and other friends and her job, but in fact had lost them *because* she was suffering from a depressive illness.

The BBC people were so charmed by Grocers' Gift that they built a replica of it in the studio, but with holes for the cameras to look through.

We realised that a series which was to go out at a peak viewing time on a Saturday on BBC 1 would lead to an avalanche of calls, so for the period from February to May 1972 I borrowed a disused Church School at Stepney, 'the Greencoat School, Hamlet of Ratcliff,' and filled it with bunk beds and desks and most important of all, fifty telephones all on the number 790 3456, which was the number used by the actors when answering the emergency 'phones in the mock-up of Grocers' Gift. The School was manned by volunteers from all over the country (only one person backed out on discovering that the two dormitories were not male and female, but smoking and non-smoking). It was bitterly cold and meals were makeshift, but as I was the only person who lived there for the whole period, it didn't matter. I still remember as we squatted, wrapped in blankets, round the television set for the first episode, the first time an actor said 'seven-nine-oh-three-four-five-six The Samaritans can I help you?' *all* the fifty 'phones rang, and as we answered each one, the person who had rung to 'see if it was real' hung up and then it rang again. After everyone's curiosity was satisfied, we began to get real calls from all over the country, and were able to put most people in touch with their local Branch but still had much befriending to do ourselves as the short-lived 'East End Annexe' of the London Branch.

Nothing in the way of publicity, before or since, has so increased the number of our callers. Small Branches reported quadrupling, and even our biggest Branches doubling, of numbers both of those seeking help and of people wanting to join us. The glamorisation inseparable from television meant that the series brought acceptable callers much more than usable volunteers.

Altogether, the exercise was such a success that we wanted the series repeated or a new series made. Unfortunately, however, people within the movement who ought to have known better had given the false impression to the BBC that 'the Samaritans didn't like it,' whereupon the tapes (which had cost £60,000 each in those days) were wiped and no further series was to be considered. Before this happened, however, the series was shown in several other countries, including Malaysia, New Zealand, Singapore and Zambia. I remember on one of my visits to our Branch in Singapore I had to address the volunteers at a meeting in the YMCA on Depression, and when I arrived they said they were going to watch some television first (there were two huge sets on the stage). I sat with Janet Lim, who had worked in the London Branch, recognised familiar music, and looked up to see on the screens NOBODY UNDERSTANDS MIRANDA by CHAD VARAH, and everyone clapped and giggled at the surprise they had for me. Malaysia had the series at the same time on a different day, and as a Muslim country where the name 'Samaritan' is meaningless, 'The Befrienders' was happily adopted by the Branch in Kuala Lumpur.

The third outstanding event towards the end of this period was the granting to us of Royal Patronage. Her Royal Highness The Duchess of Kent became Patron of The Samaritans, and it was typical of her to wish to go through the selection procedure and, if accepted, to work as a Samaritan even if only for a short time because of her many other commitments. It was my privilege to put Her Royal Highness through this procedure, part of which took place in the squalor of the Hamlet of Ratcliff School and to discover what a natural Samaritan we had been fortunate to acquire as our Patron. Working only on the telephone, for obvious reasons, no caller ever knew who '1500' really was.

The third decade

Towards the end of my 21 years as Director of the London Branch I began to feel that I must choose between it and my increasing involvement with our Branches in other parts of the world, for I couldn't do justice to both interests. Visiting Samaritans always come to London and I have always had a policy of dropping everything to make them feel welcome and to strengthen their Samaritan commitment. When Christopher Pepys died, I was allowed to take over the 'Overseas Committee' which he had briefly chaired, but I disliked the name because the people to be cherished and encouraged naturally did not think of themselves as 'overseas'. At that time, in addition to the four Branches which had helped to form the Company in 1963, we had a Branch in Calcutta because of the vision and determination of the late Bishop Lakdasa De Mel, at that time Archbishop of Calcutta and Metropolitan of the Church of India, Burma, Pakistan and Ceylon (who later as Bishop of Kurunegala inspired Sri Lanka Sumithrayo and on his deathbed showed me the deeds of land he was giving for a centre to be built in Colombo). Rhodesia had added Bulawayo and Umtali; Professor Dr Tadeusz Kielanowski had started a Branch at Gdańsk, Poland; George Appleton, then Archbishop of Perth (later Archbishop of Jerusalem) had inspired The Samaritans of Western Australia at Perth; The Very Reverend Walter Hurst, then Dean of Wellington, became the founding father in New Zealand, with Branches at that time in Wellington and Palmerston North; the Revd Gunnar Teilmann of USA had started a Branch in Singapore; and, most important of all (as it was to turn out) Jacques A. Conchon of São Paulo Brazil who, as I have mentioned earlier, decided after a visit to me in 1965 that his methods were the same as those of The Samaritans and that he would like his growing organisation to join us. In addition, Monica Dickens (later made MBE for it) was preparing our first US Branch at Boston, and there were Branches in preparation also at Bloemfontein and in Trinidad. The way forward in Europe was blocked by The Samaritans Inc. belonging to IFOTES, and in eastern Australia and South Africa by Life Line. The USA was covered by hotlines of various kinds. Only South

America and the Caribbean, Africa and most of Asia were virgin.

Samaritans from far and wide visited me and I visited them and corresponded with them, and the culmination of all this was that I invited a number of delegates to come to England for a Conference at St Stephen Walbrook on 3 September 1974 and afterwards for the Conference of The Samaritans Inc. in the University of Manchester. Jacques Conchon had had to come the previous month, for business reasons, but attending together we had a Samaritan from Hong Kong (the founder, Andrew Tu), two from India, one from Israel, one from Malaysia, two from New Zealand, two from Rhodesia, one from Singapore, two from Sweden, one from Turkey, one from Western Australia and one from the USA. They were not only of both sexes and all age groups, but of all colours of skin. They did not know one another, but they all knew me, so it wasn't surprising that when they unanimously agreed to ask The Samaritans Inc. at the approaching Conference to release them from membership and allow them to band together as a sister organisation, Befrienders International (The Samaritans Worldwide), they should have elected me President for Life. But then when it came to electing a Chairman for the next three years, none of them felt capable of taking it on, so they elected me to that too. I didn't know that in spite of all my efforts to find someone else to take over, I should be left to serve three three-year terms and only get a successor elected then (Mrs Vanda Scott) by refusing to stand again.

The delegates received a heartwarming reception from the other Samaritans at Manchester. They elected John McKechnie, the young Director at that time of The Samaritans of Western Australia, who as a lawyer was a good choice, to join me in putting the unanimous request of our 22 delegates, backed up by dozens not present including Jacques Conchon of Brazil, to the Chairman of the Samaritans Inc. He promised to discuss it with the Executive. (We did not suspect until later, when desperate efforts were made by IFOTES to claim that Befrienders International was a part of IFOTES willy-nilly, that the embarrassment of the Samaritans Inc. was caused by their membership of IFOTES, from which they were not to escape for another ten years.)

Our twenty-first anniversary

The happy ending came a couple of months later. A Council of Management meeting was held on our actual 21st anniversary, 2 November 1974, and it was resolved at that meeting that the Branches outside the British Isles should be recognised collectively as a sister organisation, bound by the same principles, under the name Befrienders International (The Samaritans Worldwide), with the right to elect their own officers, raise their own funds and authorise and control new Branches outside the British Isles, and that with the exception of the Founder, membership should be restricted to Samaritans living and working outside the British Isles, who would if coming to live in the territory of The Samaritans Inc. come under the jurisdiction of The Samaritans Inc. It was further agreed that I, having been elected as Chairman with duties too onerous to be combined with those of Director of the London Branch, should be allowed to relinquish on that day the directorship of the London Branch and should be succeeded forthwith by the Revd John Eldrid, this being the wish of the Committee of the London Branch and of myself.

It was uphill work, and for most of the following nine years I was working alone. I could not afford a secretary, and would not have been able to afford to make the extensive journeys to the Branches in my care but for the fact that a Samaritan friend who had retired because of blindness caused by diabetes, Norman M. Watkinson, supplemented what contributions I could afford to make with very generous contributions of his own. In addition, I had wonderful hospitality from Samaritans in most places I visited, so I was able to travel the equivalent of twice round the world each year more economically than most people would have believed possible.

During the 9 years before I handed over to Mrs Vanda Scott, a former Director of The Wanchai Hong Kong Samaritans who moved to Singapore when her husband's work did and later to Dallas, Texas, I saw the number of our Branches grow from 9 to about 90. Much more of this was due to Jacques Conchon and his trusty lieutenants in Brazil than to me, and other countries too became organised on a national scale so that they had their own extension committees – in addition to

Zimbabwe and Western Australia we saw BINZ in New Zealand, Sri Lanka Sumitrayo (still trying to get a third Branch off the ground), and Samsusa, The Samaritans USA, making great progress in New England, Chicago and New York, but still in only seven of the fifty-odd States.

The saddest thing for me is when, perhaps after several visits by me, a Branch appears to be flourishing and then collapses, often because some key person leaves (perhaps an expatriate moved to some other country). It is less sad when much effort and many visits still leave a place without a Branch, because 'you can't win them all' and you never know when the bread cast upon the waters will come back toasted and buttered. It has been known for a person recruited and instructed in a place that never got a Branch going, to become the initiator of a Branch in a different continent.

Zambia at one time had four Branches and was planning two more, but is now down to none, so they were right not to listen to my urging to form a national association. India is too large, and the distances between the five Branches too expensive to cover for a meaningful association to be formed. We are in Bloemfontein and Kimberley in South Africa, in Bangkok Thailand, in Lethbridge Alberta Canada and in Mexico City – all places with room for expansion. From Barbados and Trinidad we *may* spread in the Caribbean, and from Bahrain and Oman to the rest of the Arabian Gulf, from Gothenburg through Sweden, from Oporto to the rest of Portugal, and from Osaka to the rest of Japan. All we can say is that in these and other places we have people who are true Samaritans, and if their example is not followed, their neighbours and fellow-countrymen will suffer.

Meanwhile, in the British Isles our expansion has been slowing down, and as the number of Branches exceeded 180, it was clear that saturation point had almost been reached – i.e., that convenience to a few additional clients living between existing Branches would not justify recruiting from the very limited volunteer manpower in any area a sufficient number of hand-picked people to maintain a service which would be little used and would inevitably deprive other voluntary organisations.

Improving our service

Although nothing about our work had changed since the early days when we were fortunate to 'get it right', except that we were able to give befriending to more people in more places, in our third decade we learnt to analyse what we were doing and make some improvements. The process had been a particular concern of Dr George Day of the Norwich Branch and was continued by another Samaritan doctor, Dr Roy Vining of the Lowestoft Branch, who got us to improve our ways of communicating with one another about callers, of selecting and instructing volunteers with particular emphasis on the use of role play, and most important of all, the use of a simple system of lethality scoring to enable the Leaders (whom most Branches now had between the Director and the befrienders who were still free from the burden of making decisions) to arrange special care for those assessable as 'serious and immediate suicide risks'.

Reduction of the number of suicides has always been our objective. The success or otherwise of our work is to be judged solely on whether it does or does not reduce the number of suicides in the areas in which we operate. If we are not saving lives, we are failing; and it is no good giving us pats on the back for doing something else. To decrease human misery is undoubtedly a worthy endeavour, and we may be thankful for the activities in this regard of such diverse professions as comedian, restaurateur, prostitute, hairdresser, and health visitor; but *our* task is to decrease human misery in those who might, unless this were achieved, be more likely to die by their own hands. Obviously, like any other specialists, we cannot hope to be so fortunate as to encounter only those who come clearly within the realm of our specialisation. We can, however, fashion our image and publicity in such a way as to attract the highest possible proportion of potential suicides, and the lowest possible proportion of those who are not by any stretch of the imagination likely to fall into this category. Furthermore, we can firmly decline to accept any other criterion of the success of our work than the saving of those who would otherwise have killed themselves, so that when we are praised for other socially useful things we are alleged to have done, we can make it clear that this is a mere by-product, however welcome, and not an indicator of our effectiveness in the task to which we have committed ourselves. In the same way, if the quality of befriending offered by a particular Branch were poor, it would be no satisfaction to us to be told that the Branch had excellent consultants or good relationships with the medical profession, so that clients needing an expert received excellent counselling or psychiatric treatment.

In the late Seventies, desperate attempts had been made by people whose names were more than sufficiently publicised in repeated press handouts at the time to 'prove' that the fall in suicides in Britain since 1963, unique in the world, was totally unconnected with the existence, also unique, in the same country and from the same date, of a nationwide organisation, universally known and respected and trusted, which invites suicidal people to seek their help at any hour of the day or night. I am not credulous enough to believe that an organisation which at that time had over 20,000 volunteers manning 170 Centres with 1¼ million contacts a year, listening patiently and sympathetically each year to the troubles of a quarter of a million *new* 'clients', made no difference whatever to the incidence of suicide. It should be remembered that the people thus given encouragement, moral support, and (where desired) referral to medical or other experts for further help, in conditions of total acceptance and confidentiality, have been sampled by researchers and have been found to be as 'lethal' as mental hospital patients, i.e. enormously above the national suicide rate.

Some professionals are apparently unable to bear the thought that non-professionals, however numerous, well chosen and carefully supervised, can achieve anything worth while in the field of suicide prevention. In effect, they ask the general public to believe that a graph which shows the number of Samaritan Branches, clients and volunteers steadily increasing, and at the same time the number of suicidal deaths decreasing in proportion, so that an X is formed on the graph, is pure coincidence.

If we examine countries comparable to the British Isles in being Western-style industrial democracies, with excellent medical facilities, particularly casualty and resuscitation services and intensive care, we find that their standards of diagnosis and treatment are at least equal to what is found in the British Isles, but they either have no Samaritans at all, or the Samaritans are recently established and have not yet become widespread and widely used. In these countries, the suicide rate has remained steady or has risen.

Our denigrators, eccentric though their ideas of plausibility seemed to me to be, confined themselves to denying the effectiveness in suicide prevention of anything that The Samaritans or others were doing. They did not go to the lengths of making any positive suggestions as to what might usefully be done.

We are no longer bound by Durkheim's views of 1897, when study of the phenomenon of suicide led to the depressing conclusion arrived at that there was no way its incidence could be changed by trying to do so. The rate would go up in times of social disorganisation and down in time of war, and nothing else would prevent the steady rise which we now attribute to increasing urbanisation. Durkheim, genius though he was, could not be expected to envisage in his day such creatures as Samaritans, let alone their numbers and activity and widespread acceptance. He was rather in the position of a man who, if he had thought about it at all, would have 'known' that it would be impossible to recruit billions of little people with tiny syringes to draw infinitesimal drops of nectar from trillions of flowers in order to make for mankind a sweet viscous substance called honey. If he *had* thought of it, he would have 'known' that it would cost a million pounds a pound. We who can all afford to have it on our breakfast tables must not sneer at the fellow who was handicapped by never having encountered or heard of bees.

In our third decade, the fall in suicides in England and Wales tended to level out, but it is worth noting that at the same time there was a general upward tendency throughout the world and it was *still* true that no country without a busy network of Samaritan Branches had reduced its suicide rate.

Parasuicide

One worrying phenomenon was the increase in parasuicides, especially in the young. I think we have to face the fact that our listening therapy, offered at a moment's notice day or night, which is the most effective way of helping people with a moderate to high lethality, is, by its very nature, less effective with the person who is using the act of self-injury as a fairly deliberately chosen means of non-verbal communication.

It is distressing for the parasuicide and his or her family and burdensome for our casualty departments, but worst of all it is usually an *ineffective* form of communicating their need for help. There are not the resources to give all parasuicides the psychiatric or casework attention which might benefit them, and in many cases Samaritan befriending may be what they ought to have sought but didn't. The practice of some hospitals of giving to persons discharged after treatment for an act of self-injury a card in a plain envelope giving details of the local Branch of The Samaritans is probably the best answer so far devised.

In the long term, our unsung heroes and heroines who go into schools to talk about our work point to the even more satisfactory answer of teaching youngsters to communicate their distresses verbally. At the same time they can often help youngsters in their formative years to a better understanding between the sexes. If successful, this could reduce teenage pregnancies, unhappy marriages, worries about homosexuality, and the attitudes which lead to the horrors of rape.

Our panels of speakers are an important part of our publicity to attract callers and volunteers and of our fund raising.

Publicity is our life blood. We are fortunate to have been put on the right lines by David Merritt Jackson and to be guided by his successor Rex Cannon.

It is obvious that an organisation existing to cater for a small proportion of the population, consisting of people whose identities are not known, can communicate with its potential clients only by making the fullest possible use of the media: press, radio, television, advertising, posters, and such things as slogans on T-shirts worn on sponsored walks. By informing everybody, repeatedly, about the nature and purpose of the service offered, it may be hoped that those who need to avail themselves of it will become aware of it. There are, of course, exceptions to this: the isolated and elderly may be too depressed to listen to the radio or read the newspaper or may live without these, so other means have to be found of communicating with this category of people who may need our help.

However it is not merely our existence but our terms of reference which need to be publicised. It makes all the difference to the kind of people who get into contact with us whether we have in our publicity accurately conveyed what we do and what we regretfully cannot undertake.

Our Branches must be clear what they exist for and what they do not exist for, and having set our own house in order, we must then make it unmistakable in our publicity what it is that we are offering and express it in such a way as to discourage as far as possible people wasting their time and ours by coming to the wrong shop. Of course, human nature leads people who urgently want some kind of help to see a possibility of getting it where none exists. If a charity is set up to help residents of Pimlico of Irish origin and Roman Catholic faith with the school fees of their daughters, it will inevitably be approached by people who are not of Irish origin and do not live in Pimlico and have no daughters but require help in paying off their rent arrears. We must therefore not be surprised that, when an organisation offers help without making such stringent restrictions, large numbers of people should consider it worth a try. If there is a discrepancy between what the Branch says it does and what it does in practice, this will become known on the grapevine, and the latter will be believed and acted upon if it is to someone's advantage. For instance, it is no good stating clearly in a press handout that The Samaritans do not give money, as is the policy in the British Isles, if there are cases where some sentimental volunteer organises a whip round for a tramp, who proceeds to tell all his colleagues, who come swarming to this honey pot and are justifiably annoyed when turned away empty-handed. It is bound to sound hard-hearted to those who cannot concentrate to say that even giving the assembly of tramps a hot drink before sending them away would run the risk of a genuine client taking one look and turning tail, certain that he had come to the wrong shop and that all the talk about suicide prevention was eyewash.

The Samaritans are now so well known that it is taken for

granted by the media that we can be referred to without explanation. We are often delighted to find ourselves the subject of humorous cartoons, for the English poke gentle fun at the institutions they most love. I think my favourite was the one showing Humpty-Dumpty looking down at someone holding a huge frying pan invitingly and enquiring, 'Are you *sure* you're from The Samaritans?'

The danger of being a household name is that we may come to be regarded as part of 'the establishment' which would deter some of those we exist to help, and that people may see us as all-purpose doers of good, which brings to us people we cannot help and never said we could help. We need constantly to stress in our publicity, and to remind ourselves, that saving lives is a sufficiently important matter for us to try to concentrate on it to the exclusion of everything else.

The freedom to choose

There is a matter of policy which deserves mention because it must have a profound effect on the nature of the publicity we receive. Are we to be known to the general public as an organisation which respects the right of a caller who expresses the intention on the telephone of killing himself or reveals that he has already done something which will shortly lead to his death, to the point that we allow him to die without any intervention by us of a kind which he has expressly refused to agree to? Or are we to be known as an organisation which is so determined to save lives that in such circumstances it would trace calls and send ambulances or police cars round to prevent the person who wanted to commit suicide from doing so? In this dilemma our policy is different from that of our colleagues in suicide prevention centres in California and in some other parts of the United States. They say that it would be irresponsible to know that a person was in danger of death by suicide and not take effective action to prevent that person's death if any possibility of doing so could be found. We, on the other hand, take the view that we should only have to force suicide prevention on an unwilling client once, and for this to be widely publicised as it inevitably would be, to destroy the confidence that clients have in us and to reduce gradually to zero the number of persons in such a situation who would venture to telephone us. However, without making any judgment on our American colleagues, who have the responsibility of making their own policy for their own clientele and who are in a better position than we are to judge the reaction of potential clients in their area, we have to say we could not possibly bring ourselves to believe such action to be justifiable in the British Isles or in any other culture in which we find ourselves operating. The difference is that we have publicised ourselves as offering disinterested help to those who approach us, whilst still leaving the caller in charge of his own destiny, so that he has nothing whatever to lose through ringing The Samaritans. He retains his freedom to say that he is grateful for the befriending he has received, but it has not made any difference and he is still of a mind to kill himself and is now going to break contact and follow that course.

According to our beliefs, the right thing for a Samaritan volunteer who receives a call on the telephone from a caller who says either that he is intending to kill himself or that he has already done some act of self-injury which will fairly shortly lead to his death, and who refuses to give his name, address and telephone number and who does not agree to any face to face intervention by or organised by The Samaritans, is to accept the conditions laid down, and regretfully to recognise that there is no feasible alternative to this. Any attempt to impose *our* conditions can only have the result of causing the caller to hang up and leave us in a situation of being unable to resume contact with him. We must face the fact that any telephone caller has us at his mercy, in that if we do not know his telephone number we have no way of resuming contact with him if he decides to hang up on us; and even if we *do* know his telephone number, we have no guarantee that he will answer if we call.

We often explain to new volunteers that 'the client is the boss', and whether we like it or not, this is most certainly the case where the clients approach us by telephone, and not in a face to face encounter. Clearly, if a person on Flying Squad goes to meet a caller at some agreed place in the middle of the night, and then is asked to stop on a high bridge, and the caller gets out and expresses the intention of jumping over to his death, there is every excuse for the volunteer to intervene physically, and to take the view that if the caller did not wish him to do so, he would have terminated the encounter, waited until the Samaritan had driven off, and *then* jumped. The fact is that people do not commit suicide in the presence of another person, though they may make suicidal gestures, for some appeal or manipulative reason. It is a different pattern when, because the contact is only by telephone, the caller knows for certain that intervention is just not possible, except by his call being traced and police or ambulance being sent. It is our firm conviction that our constituents know perfectly well that we do not force our attentions upon those who have explicitly refused them, and that our publicity has in effect promised that we will not trace calls unless, in most exceptional circumstances, we have very good grounds for supposing that that caller wants us to do so and hopes we will do so.

Samaritan procedures are not arbitrarily imposed from on high. They represent the experience of over thirty years and a distillation of the wisdom of a very great number of volunteers who have consulted with their leaders and with one another at seminars, schools, and regional and national conferences. There should be very good reasons indeed for departing from anything enjoined by this corpus of wisdom and experience. That same humility which is the chief common characteristic of Samaritans is a safeguard against the pride which leads a person to suppose that his unconsidered opinions are of more value than the carefully considered conclusions of the organisation to which he has promised his loyalty.

The fourth decade

Our thirtieth anniversary on 2 November 1983 was marked by the position of Chairman of Befrienders International (The Samaritans Worldwide) being taken over from me by Vanda Scott. There could be no more suitable beginning for our fourth decade, which I may or may not survive, because it will be one during which all the resources of our two sister organisations must be mobilised in order to make our befriending therapy available in those parts of the world where suicide is a problem and we do not yet have Branches offering a 24-hours-a-day service.

It is evident that a young wife and mother of two small

children cannot give the same amount of time to being Chairman as I was able to give. I was able to visit Branches anywhere in the world that wanted a visit, and when not travelling, I was able to spend very extended office hours at my desk, neglecting everything else except those cases referred to me from various sources for sex therapy and counselling which could be dealt with between absences abroad. There is still a shortage of people able to deal with sexual deviations, with preorgasmic women, and with lesbians who find difficulty in accepting themselves.

The election of Vanda meant that the delegation I had tried and mostly failed to do must be done. Continental and regional representatives must play their part, and the new Constitution has made it clear who must do what, and that if the appointed person does not do it, it probably will not be done, and the callers will suffer. The same difficulty that I have already mentioned of getting Samaritans to see that 'the needs of the clients dictate' that our organisation be as efficient as we can make it has been great in the British Isles but will obviously be even greater in some parts of the world, and the sheer size of 'the rest of the world' makes regionalisation even more important than it was for The Samaritans Inc.

The separation between The Samaritans Inc. and Befrienders International was never intended to be permanent. It was made for a purpose, and there are no prizes for guessing that the purpose was to bring greater benefit to more callers in more places. This purpose has gone some way towards being achieved, but even in our most successful country, Brazil, with over 60 Branches, there is still a long way to go before the whole country is served. It may well be that the time is approaching when the constituent countries of Befrienders International will feel strong enough to request The Samaritans Inc. to join them, in order that the resources of Samaritans in the British Isles, no longer needed for setting up still more new Branches, may help Branches working under great difficulties in the less developed parts of the world.

The fact that someone other than myself is in charge should make it easier for The Samaritans Inc. to respond constructively to any such suggestion.

Within 10 days of acquiring a new Chairman, Befrienders

International and I had the great joy of seeing the chief obstacle to our spread on the continent of Europe removed. At a Council of Management meeting (held on my 72nd birthday) The Samaritans Inc. decided to withdraw from IFOTES forthwith or at the earliest permissible date. The decision was made not to benefit BI (although it would) but because continued membership appeared to The Samaritans Inc. to conflict with their principles. The sadness of substantial sums being paid to the opponents of Befriending and nothing to BI was ended, and The Samaritans Inc. has helped its sister organisation by annual grants which diminish as Befrienders International builds up its own fundraising.

Not that Samaritans in the British Isles can rest upon their laurels. There are still difficult tasks facing the organisation, one of which is to improve the proportion of the time spent by Samaritans at their Branch which is actually given to befriending callers of the kind for which the movement exists. I know that this can never be 100 per cent. There has to be time for communication and consultation within the Branch, and this is as directly related to the callers' needs as are actual befriending conversations with them, on the telephone or face to face. It is also obvious that whether callers other than those who make an appointment are neatly distributed through the day or arrive in crowds after long stretches when nothing is happening, is beyond our control. Firemen and lifeboatmen face the same problem; but whereas they ought not to light fires or cause wrecks to give themselves practice and combat boredom, we can, to some extent, use periods when nothing is happening to initiate calls to lonely people who have a telephone and have indicated that they appreciate such calls.

The chief way of increasing the amount of time spent in Samaritan befriending is by selection of callers. This may seem impossible, if not actually un-Samaritan, but it is being done to some extent at present. There is surely no Branch which hasn't found it necessary to blacklist some aggressive psychopaths, or to restrict some callers whose demands for continuous attention are good neither for themselves nor for the 'real' callers, or to limit the length of time allowed to some lonely but otherwise non-urgent regular callers, or to restrict to a particular Samaritan some particularly difficult or manipulative caller. In the extreme cases, it is not difficult for even the more sentimental volunteers to see that befriending the suicidal doesn't necessarily mean being at everyone's beck and call regardless of whether this is helpful; but what about the in-between? There are people who aren't at all in crisis, who can thoroughly enjoy a chat with a charming Samaritan, and it is not their fault if we have not instructed volunteers how to distinguish those who need befriending – but always, of course, giving the caller the benefit of any doubt.

Our excellent film, 'Can I Help You?' (16 mm in colour with sound; and videotape) in 30 minutes presents an instructive and moving account of a day in the life of a small Branch (two volunteers for all shifts except the evening with four), using professional actors who are also Samaritans. Out of a splendid cast I want to praise especially John Bennett, David Cook, Carol Gillies, Freddie Jones, Miriam Karlin and Mia Soteriou: who can forget John rebuking Carol or Miriam embracing Mia? The script was by John Bowen. The dialogue has been translated into Cantonese, Flemish, French, German, Portugese and Spanish, so that by turning the sound off and having local Samaritans read the parts, it can be understood in many non-English-speaking countries. Used in this way in Mandarin, members of crisis lines not affiliated to us are trained in Taiwan. The film has received some unjust criticism, e.g. of a scene in which some callers were awaiting attention in a waiting room. (Would they have been better waiting in the street?) We all know it would be ideal if a caller could always be seen immediately, and surprisingly often he is, but it is a good thing people who think we should always have a crowd of volunteers waiting in case there's a rush, are not in charge of Branches. It is a good thing, too, that Samaritans are not put in the charge of anyone who does not see that befriending is a relationship and that those who are so emotionally immature and undeveloped that they can neither give nor receive love are quite literally unbefriendable.

The film 'Can I help you?' replaced an earlier one in which the distressed caller was played by that excellent actress Sandy Ratcliff, now appearing regularly in the BBC's successful

EastEnders, and the Samaritan who befriended her by the actress Suzan Cameron who was at that time my secretary.

Now the Children's Film Unit has made an excellent video for us, splendidly scripted and acted. It was received with acclaim by those of the 1200 Samaritans at the annual Conference in the University of York in September 1986 who were privileged to see it. Only one line given to the actress Pamela Blackwood was rejected as un-Samaritan – 'Try not to worry too much, won't you?'

It was at this Conference that I was able to announce to my fellow-Samaritans that I was with them for the last time, as I had decided to retire from everything except being historically the Founder on 2 November 1986, on completing a third of a century. The Samaritans, I said, were 33 years old and even Befrienders International on the point of becoming a teenager, so they no longer needed a Daddy. St Stephen Walbrook, I told them, had been restored over nine years at a cost of over a million pounds, and embellished by an altar carved from Roman travertine marble by the late Henry Moore. As its Rector, the least I could do was to devote my whole time to its service, knowing that the movement to which I had given most of my life would continue and grow.

So we end where we began, with an approach to the problems of the suicidal people in our society which is fimly based on supplying their needs as ascertained by questioning them and observation of them, and constantly checking the validity of this as the years go by, and learning from experience. An American tourist visiting an Oxford College told the gardener he'd like a lawn like the one in the quad. 'Easy, zur,' said the man, 'ye sows. Then ye mows and ye rolls and ye *weeds*. And ye keeps on for three 'undred year. It's easy.'

We haven't yet been going for 300 years but already we know that our befriending is preventing suicide. We also know that amongst the lives we have saved from being wasted are our own.

Befriending is offered for the benefit of the client, and is limited to the duration and extent of the client's need – not the volunteer's.

Depressed people may be temporarily incapable of holding up their end of a mutual friendship; family and friends get bored, impatient, fed up. Samaritan befriending offers a one-sided, temporarily dependent friendship to people who might not be chosen as friends apart from their need. The lack of mutuality allows the client the luxury of being completely self-absorbed; and the Samaritan gives his full undivided attention without expecting equal time in return.

Is is a therapeutic, not a social, relationship.

The client is offered simple, uncomplicated support, and remains free to make his own decisions, reject help, break contact – even take his own life without fear of unwanted interference.

While this lack of mutuality frees the client, it can be hard on the volunteer. Sometimes befriending is a tedious, thankless job and we feel worried and sad and helpless and inadequate. The clients didn't ask us to join The Samaritans, and they are not obliged to make us feel worthwhile.

SALLY CASPER
in *Answers to Suicide*

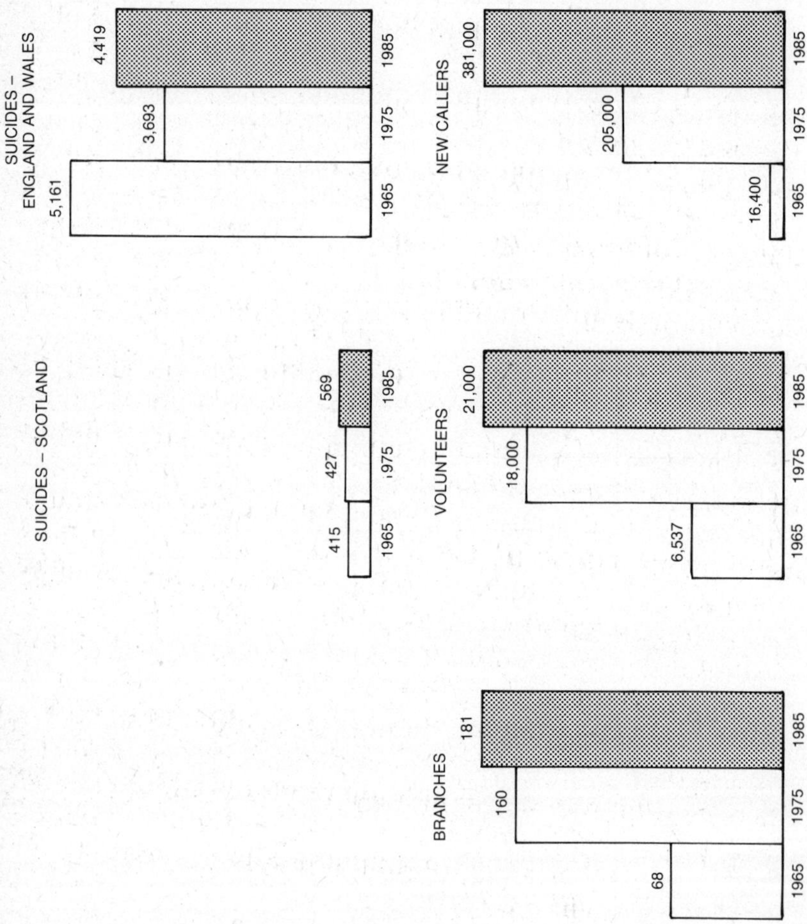
SUICIDES – ENGLAND AND WALES
5,161
3,693
4,419
1965
1975
1985
SUICIDES – SCOTLAND
415
427
569
1965
1975
1985
NEW CALLERS
16,400
205,000
381,000
1965
1975
1985
VOLUNTEERS
6,537
18,000
21,000
1965
1975
1985
BRANCHES
68
160
181
1965
1975
1985

Suicides and the numbers of Samaritan Branches in England and Wales 1959 – 85

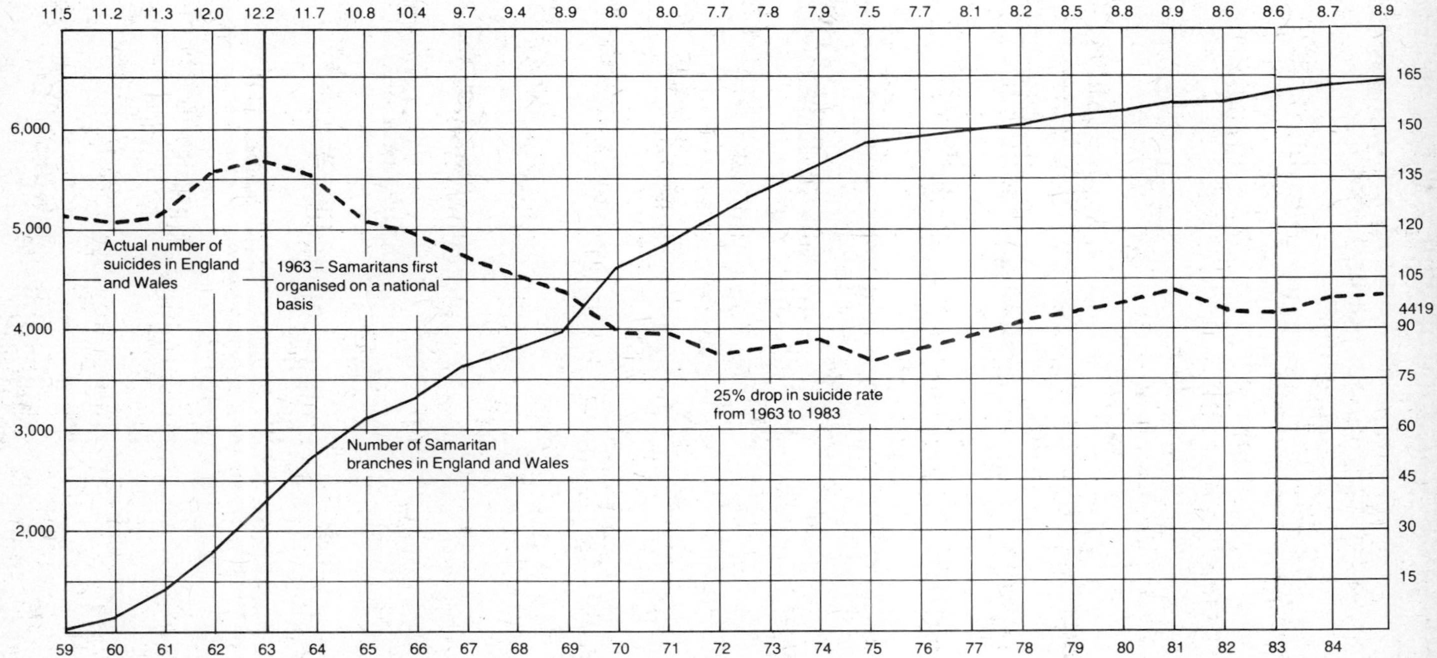

Year	1974	1975	1976	1977	1978	1979	1980	1981	1982	1983	1984	1985
Suicides in England and Wales	3,891	3,689	3,813	3,976	4,019	4,195	4,314	4,424	4,279	4,279	4,315	4,419
New callers in the British Isles	192,184	204,978	209,518	229,970	250,740	273,525	309,742	314,740	319,117	328,656	358,500	383,007
Samaritans in the British Isles	18,022	18,539	19,294	19,801	20,131	20,329	20,943	21,021	20,004	20,101	20,269	21,313

How the Samaritans Help

The Samaritans offer a free and completely confidential emergency and befriending service 24 hours a day, seven days a week including Christmas and all bank holidays.

The Samaritans in the British Isles have 187 centres and over 21,000 carefully selected and prepared volunteers who give nearly three million hours of work at these centres every year – 8,000 hours every day.

In 1985 the Samaritans received over two million calls and visits which is an increase of 23 per cent since 1982. This represents nearly 6,000 calls a day or one call every 15 seconds. Those making contact for the first time exceeded 383,000 – an increase of 20 per cent since 1982.

The Principles of The Samaritans

the samaritans

THE PRINCIPLES AND PRACTICES

SEVEN PRINCIPLES

1. The primary aim of The Samaritans is to be available at any hour of the day or night to befriend those passing through personal crises and in imminent danger of taking their own lives.

2. The Samaritans also seek to alleviate human misery, loneliness, despair and depression by listening to and befriending those who feel that they have no one else to turn to who would understand and accept them.

3. A caller does not lose the freedom to make his own decisions, including the decision to take his own life, and is free to break contact at any time.

4. The fact that a person has asked the help of The Samaritans, together with everything he has said, is completely confidential within the organisation unless permission is freely given by the caller for all or a part of such information to be

communicated to someone outside the organisation. A Samaritan volunteer is not permitted to accept confidences if a condition is made that not even the Director should be informed of them.

5. Samaritan volunteers in befriending callers will be guided and actively supported by experienced leaders who will have the advice, when required, of professional consultants.

6. In appropriate cases the caller will also be invited to consider seeking professional help in such fields as medicine and social work, and material help from other agencies.

7. Samaritan volunteers are forbidden to impose their own convictions or to influence callers in regard to politics, philosophy or religion.

SEVEN PRACTICES

1. Samaritan volunteers are carefully selected and prepared by the local Branch in which they are to serve.

2. The Samaritans are available at all hours to callers, and may be contacted (anonymously if desired) by telephone or personal visit, or by letter.

3. When a caller is believed to be in danger of suicidal action, the Samaritan is particularly encouraged to ask the caller's permission for contact to be maintained during the crisis.

4. Samaritans offer longer-term befriending of callers where appropriate, while recognising that the Branch may from time to time have to set limits.

5. Samaritans listen to those concerned about the welfare of another person, and, if satisfied that the third person is despairing, depressed or suicidal, may discreetly offer befriending.

6. Samaritans are normally known to callers only by a forename and contacts by callers made only through the Branch centre.

7. Samaritan Branches are banded together in a legally constituted Association whose Council of Management represents all the Branches and reserves to itself the appointment of the person in charge of each Branch.

Only the Council of Management, which is responsible for the work of The Samaritans in the United Kingdom, the Isle of Man, the Channel Islands and the Republic of Ireland, can revise these principles and practices, or authorise Branches to depart from them.

BEFRIENDERS INTERNATIONAL

– The Samaritans Worldwide

Befrienders all over the world made suggestions during the drafting in 1981 of the Seven Principles and Seven Practices, based on the Founder's Twenty Principles, and found the final form acceptable, with minor emendations which were unanimously incorporated when the Constitution (drafted in 1984) was finalised and agreed. In Principle no. 6 'may' was preferred to 'will'; Practice no. 2, because callers in some countries do not use the telephone, and volunteers are hard to find, was re-worded:

2. Samaritans aim to be available at all hours, and may be contacted by personal visit or by letter or (anonymously if desired) by telephone.

We all desire to have every person who has ever been accepted as a Samaritan anywhere in the world identifiable by a Christian name or forename or Samaritan nickname plus a unique number made up of their number in their Branch, the number of the Branch in the country in which it is situated, and the number allocated to that country – all three usually in order of seniority. Therefore the BI (SW) version of Practice no. 6 reads:

6. Samaritans are normally known to callers only by a first name and Samaritan volunteer number and contacts by callers are made only through the Branch centre.

The final paragraph reads: '*Only the Council of Management, which is responsible for the work of The Samaritans everywhere in the world except in the U.K., the Channel Islands, the Isle of Man and the Republic of Ireland can revise these principles and practices, or authorise Branches to depart from them.*'

Ten Commonalities of Suicide and their Implications for Response★ – EDWIN S. SHNEIDMAN

The driving idea behind this paper is the common-sense belief that effective therapy depends on assessment which is accurate and that accurate assessment depends on meaningful definition. When definitions are inadequate, it is unlikely that effective remediations can be found. The focus of this paper is committed suicide, specifically the prevention of suicide.

The main question is: what is *common* to committed suicide? That is: what are the interesting, relevant dimensions, the *common* features or characteristics of suicide that can be delineated from a common-sense point of view?

An advertent, conscious effort was made to formulate a new theory of suicide by employing a new approach to the task, trying to come to grips with the topic without leaning on either of the two giants in this field, Durkheim and Freud, or simply advancing some variation on the traditional sociological or psychodynamic approaches. Three fields were held to be propaedeutic to a new suicidology: cosmology (a view of the world); personology (an understanding of the person); and systems theory (a synthesis of disparate types of information). The principal textbooks of this new proposed approach are, respectively, Stephen Peppers's *World Hypotheses* (1942), Henry A. Murray's *Explorations in Personality* (1938) and James G. Miller's *Living Systems* (1978).

Here are some salient characteristics – *the ten commonalities* – of suicide.

1. *The common purpose of suicide is to seek a solution.*

First of all, suicide is not a random act. It is never done

★ From *Definition of Suicide* (NY: Wiley, 1985).

pointlessly or purposelessly. It is a way out of a problem, a dilemma, a bind, a challenge, a difficulty, a crisis, an unbearable situation. It has an inexorable logic and impetus of its own. It is *the* answer – the only available answer – to a real puzzler: how to get out of this? what to do? Every suicide has as its purpose the seeking of a solution to a perceived problem that is generating intense suffering. To understand what a suicide is about, one must know the problems it was intended to solve.

2. *The common goal of suicide is cessation of consciousness.*
In a curious and paradoxical way, suicide is both a moving toward and a moving away from something; the something that it is moving toward, the common practical goal of suicide is the complete stopping of one's flow of consciousness of unendurable pain as the solution to life's painful and pressing problems. ('Death' is a by-product.) The moment that the idea of the possibility of stopping consciousness occurs to the anguished mind as the answer or the way out in the presence of unusual constriction and elevated perturbation and high lethality – the three essential ingredients of suicide – then the igniting spark has been added and the active suicidal scenario has begun.

3. *The common stimulus (or information input) in suicide is unendurable psychological pain.*
If cessation is what the suicidal person is moving toward, *pain* is what that person is seeking to escape. In any close analysis, suicide is best understood as a combined movement toward cessation and as a movement away from unendurable pain, unacceptable anguish. No one commits suicide out of joy; no suicide is born out of exaltation. It is psychological pain of which we are speaking; metapain; the pain of feeling pain. The clinical rule is: reduce the level of suffering (perturbation) – often just a little – and the individual will choose to live.

4. *The common stressor in suicide is frustrated psychological needs.*
Suicide is best understood not as an unreasonable act – every suicide seems logical to the person who commits it given that person's major premises, style of syllogizing, and constricted

focus – but rather as a reaction to frustrated psychological needs. A suicide is committed because of thwarted or unfulfilled needs. Needs are the very colour and texture of our inner life. There are many pointless deaths, but there is never a needless suicide. Redress the frustrated needs and the suicide will not occur.

5. *The common emotion is helplessness-hopelessness.*

At the beginning of life the common emotion is probably randomised general excitement. In the suicidal state it is a pervasive feeling of helplessness-hopelessness: 'There is nothing that I can do (except to commit suicide) and there is no one who can help me (with the pain that I am suffering).' Historically – in the twentieth century, that is – hostility was deemed to be the basic emotion in suicide. But today suicidologists know that there are other deep basic emotions: shame, guilt, frustrated dependency. But underlying all of these is that emotion of active, impotent ennui, the feeling of helplessness-hopelessness.

This generalised emotion shows itself as elevated perturbation. Experience has taught us the important fact that it is neither possible nor practical in an individual who is highly lethal and highly perturbed to attempt to deal with the lethality directly, either by moral suasion, confrontatory interpretations, exhortation or whatever. (It does not work any better in suicide than it does in alcoholism.) The most effective way to reduce elevated lethality is by doing so indirectly, that is, by reducing the elevated perturbation. The therapist acts as ombudsman for the patient, promoting his or her interests and welfare. The goal is to reduce the real-life pressures that are driving up the person's sense of perturbation. The basic principle is this: to decrease lethality one does what needs to be done to pull the level of perturbation down – and with that action brings down the active level of lethality.

6. *The common internal attitude toward suicide is ambivalence.*

Freud brought to our attention the unforgettable psychological truth that transcends the Aristotelian appearance of the neatness of logic. Something can be *both* A and non-A. We can both like and dislike the same person; we can both love and hate a spouse, a child. On important issues we are often of two minds. The prototypical suicidal state is one in which an individual cuts his throat and cries for help at the same time, and is genuine in both of these acts. Ambivalence is the common internal attitude towards suicide: to feel that one has to do it and, simultaneously, to yearn (and even plan) for rescue and intervention. The therapist uses this ambivalence and plays for time so that the affect, rather than the bullet, is discharged.

7. *The common cognitive state is constriction.*

Suicide is not best understood as a psychosis, a neurosis or a character disorder, but is more accurately conceptualised as a more-or-less transient psychological constriction of affect and intellect. Synonyms for constriction are a tunnelling or focussing or narrowing of the range of options usually available to *that* individual's consciousness when the mind is not panicked into dichotomous thinking: either some specific (almost magical) total solution *or* cessation; all or nothing; *Caesar aut nihil*; the range of choices has narrowed to two – not very much of a range. The usual life-sustaining images of loved ones are not disregarded: worse, they are not even within the range of what is in the mind. Any attempt at rescue or remediation has to deal almost from the first with the pathological constriction.

This fact, that suicide is committed by individuals who are in a special constriction condition leads us to suggest that no one should ever commit suicide while disturbed or suicidal. It takes a mind capable of scanning a range of options greater than two to make a decision as important as taking one's life. It is vital to counter the suicidal person's constriction-of-thought by attempting to widen the mental blinkers and to increase the number of options beyond the two options of either having some magical resolution or being dead.

8. *The common action in suicide is escape (egression).*

Egression is a person's intended departure from a region of distress. Egressions include running away from home, quitting a job, deserting an army, leaving a spouse. Suicide is the ultimate egression. We must distinguish between the harmless wish to get away and the need to end it all, to stop it for real. The point of suicide is a radical and permanent change of scene; the action to effect it is to leave. We prevent egressions by blocking exits – e.g. obtaining the gun – or reducing the person's need to egress.

9. *The common interpersonal act in suicide is communication of intention.*

Perhaps the most interesting finding from large numbers of retrospective psychological autopsies of suicidal deaths is that in almost every case there were clear clues to the impending lethal event. Individuals intent on committing suicide, albeit ambivalently-minded about it, consciously or unconsciously emit signals of distress, whimpers of helplessness, pleas for response, opportunities for rescue in the usually dyadic interplay that is an integral part of the suicidal drama. It is a sad and paradoxical thing to note that the common interpersonal act of suicide is not hostility, nor rage or destruction, not even withdrawal, but communication of intention. Everyone in suicidology now knows the usual clues, verbal and behavioural. The recognition of these clues is indispensable as one way among many of preventing suicide.

10. *The common consistency in suicide is with life-long coping patterns.*

In suicide we are initially thrown off the scent because suicide is an act, by definition, which that individual has never done before so there is no precedent. And yet there are deep consistencies with life-long coping patterns. We must look to previous episodes of disturbance, to the individual's capacity to endure psychological pain, to the penchant for constriction and dichotomous thinking, for earlier paradigms of egression.

A definition of suicide which emerges from this view is as follows: currently in the Western world, suicide is a conscious act of self-induced annihilation, best understood as a multidimensional malaise in a needful individual who defines an issue for which the suicide is perceived as the best solution.

All of this is about suicide, i.e. committed suicide. Parasuicide is another topic and has its own common characteristics and its own implications for response, treatment and therapy.

Working with highly suicidal persons borrows from the goals of befriending and crisis intervention: not to take on and attempt to ameliorate the individual's entire personality structure and cure all the neurosis but simply to keep the person *alive*. This is the *sine qua non* without which all other psychotherapy and efforts to be helpful could not have the opportunity to function.

Most people would agree that the best prevention is primary prevention; an ounce of prevention is worth a pound of cure. The primary prevention of suicide lies in education. The route is through teaching one another and that large, amorphous group known as the public that suicide can happen to anyone, that there are discernible desiderata (if one but has the perspicacity to see and hear them when they occur) and that help is available. Perhaps the main task lies in the dissemination of information, especially about the clues to suicide: in schools, in the workplace, through the public media. In the end, effective prevention of suicide is everybody's business.

They told me, Heraclitus, they told me you were dead:
They brought me bitter news to hear and bitter tears to shed.
I wept as I remembered how often you and I
Had tired the sun with talking and sent him down the sky.
And now that thou art lying, my dear old Carian guest,
A handful of grey ashes, long, long ago at rest,
Still are thy pleasant voices, thy nightingales, awake:
For death he taketh all away, but them he cannot take.

WILLIAM CORY, *after Callimachus*

Psychological problems – DORIS ODLUM

We all have difficulty at times in knowing the kind of people we are dealing with and what really their basic personality and mental state is. It is in the case of people whose mental state is somewhat unstable that I think we find our greatest difficulty, because obviously the Samaritans are not trained in the diagnosis of mental disorder of any form, and the milder forms are peculiarly difficult sometimes to diagnose so that Samaritans know what they are handling. Obviously I am not suggesting that they can hope to do anything very skilled in the way of diagnosis, but at least they can learn enough to *know* when they are dealing with something which they cannot deal with. When to let go or when to pass on is a thing that requires great wisdom and experience, and sometimes a good deal of courage and modesty. It is awfully easy to feel that one does not want to be beaten by a case. I often have to tell my social workers and my junior psychiatrists that they must not feel this way at all; that it is not a shameful thing; because there are cases that only the most expert people can hope to deal with and even they cannot deal with all of them. We too know that we are helpless in certain cases to do much more than just comfort. We cannot hope to cure, we may not even be able to palliate to any great extent. And we have, of course, to accept this without feelings of guilt. It is important for us all to learn this: to know where we get out, and where we are right in getting out. It does take a good deal of practice and also humility and courage, especially with these people who are in some way mentally different from the rest of us.

Now the subjects of depression and some forms of psychopathic personality are dealt with elsewhere in this book, but the type of cases of what we call the psychotic degree, that is, the people who are suffering from a real form of mental illness which affects the whole balance of the mind, include other things than these. One is schizophrenia, a name with which I think everybody is familiar today; but schizophrenia is a complicated thing. It is not just one condition: it has many forms and facets, and it is not easy to say exactly what are the characteristics of the schizophrenic person; or perhaps we should say the schizoid person, because there are many people who have the schizoid type of background who are not necessarily suffering from the illness which we call schizophrenia in a developed form.

One of the hallmarks of these people is that as soon as one comes into contact with them, one has the feeling of strangeness, of a barrier, that somehow one cannot quite get through. One has a feeling of what I always call 'the dark vacuum' between oneself and them; so that though they appear to be wanting one's help, though they come to one for help, there is always this feeling that somehow they are withdrawn from one and that one cannot quite get over to them. Now this is a sort of instinctive feeling that one has, but I think it is a true one, and whenever one has that in relation to anyone who is asking for help, I would accept it as probably meaning that there is this basis of schizoid attitude behind it. It is very important to realise this because it will affect, or should affect, one's approach to them very materially. It means that one will very soon find oneself out of one's depth with them: that they may appear to be co-operative, to be wanting to take part in whatever assistance one is prepared to give them, and do their share, but the odds are that they will not be able to. The odds are that they will appear to accept what one says and what one does, and then one will find that nothing of the kind has happened, that they have not pursued it. They have not had the continuity of purpose or the sense of reality to carry out the course that one has perhaps agreed upon, and therefore one will find that one is not getting anywhere with them.

It is important to know this, otherwise one can get very distressed. One feels that one is failing, or that one does not know where one is, and I think one must not try to do too much where one feels this strange barrier. And not infrequently one will find, especially with the younger type of schizophrenic, that these people also have a great deal of hysteria. I am going to talk about hysteria later, but I must mention it here because the hysterical overlay is very common in young schizophrenics and they may appear to be self-dramatizing. They may appear to be showing off, posing – and indeed they very often are because many schizophrenics do live in a world of dream of their own, in which they are, in fact, acting a role for their own benefit and that of an imaginary audience. Sometimes this role is one which gives them great satisfaction – it does not give anybody else any satisfaction but it gives them some – and they are happy in it. But very often this role is one which to them is extremely frightening. They have the feeling that the world is against them, that they are pursued by enemies or that people are not appreciating them, and they can become very hostile, and as we know, one of the characteristics of schizophrenia is a sudden impulse, so that they may do very impulsive and unexpected things. So one has always to be on one's guard when meeting anybody with whom one has this kind of feeling of strangeness or remoteness or that they are not quite in touch with reality.

A type which is very closely allied to schizophrenia that we meet very often in the world we call the paranoid. These are people who live in a world where they are suspicious, hostile, believing that everybody is an enemy or ready to be an enemy, very often believing that people think they are bad and very often, especially with women, that they are sexually bad. It is extraordinary how one gets women of a perfectly blameless life believing that the world thinks they are immoral, or that they have immoral ideas, and so one gets this attitude of hostility and resentment towards the world. They are very difficult to deal with. Not infrequently they want one to change the rest of the world to suit them – and this, of course, is not easy. At first one is the new thing, and we all know that with new people, like new drugs, patients are apt to make a rather wonderful improvement for a short time. It is very easy to say to oneself, 'Ah, you see, I have succeeded where everybody else has failed. This person has told me something which they have never told anybody else.' One gets a nasty shock later because one finds they have told *everybody* else. But for a time one might very easily be deceived into thinking that one has some white magic that nobody else has got. I had this when I was young. I had to be cured of it by some very bitter experiences. We all have it, of course. For the time being one is the only person who has understood them, the one person who is going to perform all the magic that is going to take away their fears and their hostility and make everything come right. Unfortunately this does not last. Familiarity definitely breeds contempt, and before very long one will join the ranks of the enemies. I think one must understand this, otherwise one might become depressed and distressed and feel that in some way one has failed. Well, one has not. One is just dealing with a type of personality in whom this is practically inevitable. It may be that they will still retain some slight affection and confidence in one, but one will certainly not fill the bill that they had hoped one would fill and I think one had better recognise that right at the start. It is often very difficult when one is faced with a person who appears to be so charming, so delightful, so attractive and who gradually, as the story unfolds, begins to tell one of their family who have never understood them, how their husband did not really appreciate them, how the children have failed them, their bosses have not done well by them. In fact, one begins to see that the whole world has failed them all along the line and then gradually it is borne in on one that they are the paranoid type. But one can easily be deceived into believing that their family has been very cruel to them and one can go around in a state of righteous indignation, make a lot of trouble, and make a fool of oneself, if one is not careful, as we have all done – I have done it myself, so I know quite well that one can do that.

These are the two main types which one is likely to have to deal with. One must not expect to be able to do very much for them, and must realise that it may be necessary to invoke the help of people more experienced and skilled in the situation than oneself. Of course, the difficulty will be that they are very unwilling to let one invoke help. One cannot go to a doctor, one cannot go to anybody, about a patient without their consent. This would be a breach of confidence. This is a thing we have all got to be awfully careful about. We must not do that, although we might feel (and we might be right) that it would be for their own good if we did. But still, this question of confidence, with Samaritans as with the doctor, is sacred. It is as sacred as the confessional, I always feel, and one should never, never break it. For although one might feel that good will come of it, in fact it never does. It always ends in trouble in the long run. So it may be that they will refuse to let one give them the help that one feels one could acquire for them by going to a doctor, going to a social worker, going to some agency or other. They will not consent and therefore one's hands are tied, and one feels, 'Well, what can I do?' and one cannot do very much. Even so, it may still be possible to befriend them up to a point, because these people are naturally very friendless and they are unable to make a relationship of love with others. This is one of the things they cannot do: they cannot love others. Therefore their own lives are very empty of love, and this they feel. They feel that everybody is rejecting them. The truth is that it is they who are doing the rejecting, but they do not see that, and therefore they are sometimes much helped by the fact that somebody does stick to them and is not put off too badly by their hostility and by the fact that they just do not co-operate. So sometimes one can befriend them when one cannot do anything else; but here again it may often be necessary to ask some senior person to give one some guidance.

Now we come to the group of people who are suffering from some kind of what we call neurosis. The essential difference between neurosis and psychosis is that the people with the neuroses have a good deal of insight, whereas the people with the psychoses, the schizophrenics and the paranoids, and those depressives who are suffering from the endogenous type of depression, have no insight at all. That is one of the characteristics of the illness. They cannot realise that they are ill; they cannot realise that it is they who are 'different' and they feel that it is everyone else that is different. But the neurotics are very much aware of their differences. It is one of the things that distress them so much. They feel they are different from the rest of the world. When I worked in a general hospital – one of the hospitals of the Royal Free Group among others – I was seeing people who were not mentally ill, but who were emotionally disturbed, predominantly, and we found that about seventy-five per cent of our patients were suffering from some sort of anxiety state. This is the commonest form of neurosis that one gets. There are between thirty and forty per cent of the ordinary population who are in some ways rather more vulnerable and rather more sensitive than the remaining sixty per cent. These people seem to be more vulnerable to life in every way: they are more aware of themselves, more self-conscious; they are more conscious of the effects of other people upon them; they are more inclined to get worried and anxious and to find life difficult, than the other sixty per cent, whom we might call the tough. And they are a type who are very unwelcome to the other sixty per cent. The tough just do not understand them: they cannot see why they are like this, and they are often very impatient, and hostile, and even unkind to them. These more vulnerable types are largely people who are what one would call 'anxiety-prone'. They are a very fine type as a rule; the majority of them are a very good type indeed. They are the salt of the earth; they are carrying the burden of the community; they are highly conscientious; they include the perfectionists, the self-drivers, who not only drive themselves but everybody else incidentally; and they are people who cannot tolerate anything below the standards they themselves have set up for themselves and for others. One can see that if one gets this attitude, the stage is set for a great deal of difficulty in the world, because if one is always feeling the need to be on one's toes, to do that little bit more, and one dare not sit back and take things easy, one is set for a good deal of trouble. These people, although they can love very deeply and frequently do, and are good parents, good at their work – very good in every way – are often people who are touchy and difficult to live with. So we get a certain number of them because they are rather at odds with their environment and their personal relationships are very often upset. Samaritans get quite a number of these coming to them, I know. Very often it is their husbands or wives that they cannot get on with, or their children, especially their adolescent children, or it is their jobs they cannot get on with, a boss or a colleague upsets them. A certain feeling of tension, of apprehension, is their hall-mark. One can see it the moment a person of that type comes into the room. One can tell that they are that type, and one knows that one is going to have difficulty in helping them just because they are going to find it frightfully difficult to change in any way this rigid standard that they have set up for themselves. They are worriers, and they feel that they *ought* to worry; they feel that it would be in some way wrong and even dangerous not to worry. They feel that they dare not and should not relax. They have a quite unreasonable feeling of responsibility for what is happening, and they very often feel that nobody can do it as well as themselves. They are essentially the do-it-yourself type. And they very often overdo it: they cannot delegate, they cannot share with others. This makes it harder for themselves and, of course, it makes it rather hard for others too. A Samaritan will often get a husband coming and saying, 'Oh, my wife, she never stops cleaning the house. I can't get her to stop. She is always doing entirely unnecessary things, and when I ask her not to do so much or to have more help, or something or the other, she always says, "Oh, you don't understand, nobody can do it the proper way",' and so she wears herself out, and then she is irritable and troublesome and disagreeable, and here one gets a bad picture which can lead to a very unhappy family relationship, and a broken home in some cases. So these too are people that a Samaritan has to understand.

They are not of course people who want jollying along. They are not people who want scolding, either. Both methods will have been tried on them by a good many other people, but they are not successful. I think it is by making them realise that one does understand how they feel, and that one appreciates their very fine qualities, and by trying to coax them into taking a less tense, a less rigid, a less perfectionist attitude, that one can help them most. It is not easy, but I think one can do a lot with these people; one really can help them, and one can very often help their families too, by understanding their situation. Now, it is perhaps a little off the Samaritan beat to mention that these are the type of people who produce all kinds of functional physical conditions which we call psychosomatic: the sort that is very often affecting their digestion. (It is, of course, quite common for anxiety and tension to affect the digestive tracts.) Such people get headaches; they very often get some kind of skin rash when they are upset; if they have got a tendency to asthma, they will get an attack of asthma. There are many ways in which this anxiety-prone type express their anxiety through their bodies. They seem to have a peculiar *rapport* between their minds and bodies, which makes the body respond very quickly to any kind of emotional distress. This is, of course, wholly unsatisfactory, because it only exaggerates their problems. It does not in any way alleviate or do away with the psychological problem: it just increases it, because they now have a physical problem to cope with as well, and the two reinforce each other. We, as doctors, I may say, find these people difficult to assess and often extremely difficult to help. Samaritans do not have to do anything about the physical condition of such people, but some of the physical complaints which they suffer from are very strongly related to emotional distress, to a constant state of tension and anxiety. I may just say, *en passant*, that one has to be terribly careful as a doctor not to play on this string too hard because one can, if one is not very careful, assume that everything a patient of this type is suffering from is of psychological origin or psychologically increased, and one might be on a false and dangerous scent. But this is more a doctor's problem than a Samaritan's – although these people will often come to a Samaritan saying that their doctors are unsympathetic and do not understand them, and that they have all sorts of complaints which the doctors pooh-pooh and more or less disregard and just treat with sedatives or palliatives and never get really down to the problem.

Unfortunately, the general practitioner today has never been trained in handling people and their problems. The rapid increase in medical science in the last fifty years has made it almost inevitable that the years of training should be entirely devoted to increases in scientific knowledge, and our real approach to our patients as people has been neglected. Now there is a very strong feeling abroad that this is wrong, and we are trying to remedy it. The medical schools are thinking very seriously about this problem and it is to be hoped that in twenty or thirty years' time, I am afraid not much before that, the general practitioner will have a rather different approach to people. But in the meantime Samaritans are going to have a lot of people come to them, who say that they are not getting the help they want from the doctors.

Another type that we get are much fewer but with a very high nuisance value: those we call the hysterics.

Hysterical symptoms are quite different from the psychosomatic ones I have been talking about, associated with anxiety. They affect quite different aspects of the body and the mind. They affect part of the body which is concerned with the voluntary muscles and with the special senses. And they affect it in such a way that they provide an escape route, by developing hysterical blindness or voicelessness or deafness or inability to walk or inability to do something else which at least lets one out. They are not the same type as the anxiety-prone. They are much more self-indulgent; they are much more self-dramatising; they get out from under by this method, instead of facing up to it and fighting through it as anxiety-prone people do. But in fact they are not such good personality types and they are much more difficult to deal with. An hysteric is simply not prepared to make the effort to co-operate, which, after all, is essential if one is going to get anywhere. As long as a patient comes demanding a magic, he is not going to get anywhere and neither is the Samaritan and this we have to realise. It is important to know the kind of person one is dealing with and what, in fact, they are demanding from one, what they are prepared to put into the situation with one's help or with the help of others.

There is also a type which I should have referred to in association with the anxiety-prone, because they are very closely related to them and often one gets the two together: this is the obsessional type. People who are always chewing over whatever has happened. They cannot get away from it. Every problem assumes larger and larger proportions; whatever it is, they are always obsessed by it; they just cannot get it out of their minds. The obsessionals are difficult to help because of this. This is their whole personality trend, towards keeping on and on and on with the thing and working it over and over again emotionally and not being able to get it out of their system. They talk it over with all and sundry and the more they talk about it the worse they are. On the other hand, they feel this compulsive desire to talk about it and to think about it and in some ways, I suppose, one can help them a little by listening, though I think it does not do them any good to keep going to different people and whipping themselves up emotionally about it. These are people with whom Samaritans can have quite some difficulty, but I think in some cases they can help them quite considerably.

These are the main types. Of course one gets people who are suffering from frank delusions and hallucinations, or who are excitable, manic. But these are not so common; they may come into one's office in a state of complete mental disturbance, as of course can happen from time to time, but they are obviously not cases that one can handle oneself at all. Why, though, do they come to the Samaritans? Why do they not go to the agencies that exist? Here, I think, one gets a clue to a common factor in the personality of practically all the people who come to one. This is that, in some way, they are afraid of, and a little hostile to, anything that they could regard as authority, because they feel they will be despised and thought rather foolish and inadequate if they go to them. I think the reason is that they will be treated as just a case and regarded as a cog in the machine; and, of course, there is unfortunately a certain element of truth in their fear, one must admit. This is where I feel that the Samaritans are playing such a wonderful role because they have none of the institutional stigma. They are not an organisation in the same sense as the official organisations, and every person is a person to the Samaritans.

This essay was published at greater length in *The Samaritans* (1965). She 'being dead yet speaketh'.

(Hebrews xi, 4)

Crisis – GEORGE SPAUL

The Samaritans is one of the very few organisations able to deal with personal crises at the time of occurrence. Numerous organisations deal very effectively with special kinds of crisis, but the Samaritans offer a crisis service – which in availability and organisation is exactly what is required. Those who are professionally associated with the organisation work with it to increase the effectiveness of the advantages it has.

There are three types of crisis:

1. Biological
2. Environmental
3. Adventitious

These classes are not clearly differentiated and often examples are mixed, but for clarity let us say:

1. *Biological crises* are inevitable in the nature of man:
   Growth crises – e.g. weaning and puberty
   Illness in general (none of us can hope to escape illness)
   Loss of function through age
   Pregnancy and childbirth

Biological crises because inevitable *should* be prepared for through an enlightened education which would reduce their impact, making the successful resolution almost universal.

2. *Environmental crises* are not quite so inevitable. In this group the whole area of personal relations is involved in the production of crisis:
   Bereavement
   Marriage

Retirement
Migration

In this class there is often an element of personal choice, and always a relationship involved. It is the area with which psychiatrists and Samaritans are most involved.

3. *Adventitious crises* are basically due to unlucky chance:
Injury
Unemployment
Disasters – flood, fire, earthquake, famine, etc.

Crisis resolution

The process of *crisis resolution* has been studied in detail, particularly in terms of disaster and migration, but the work done in these circumstances is also applicable to the more individual crises with which we more commonly deal.

Clinically there is one characteristic of the whole period of crisis resolution and it is so important that almost all writers and original researchers comment on it. It is the *openness of the personality* at these times. There are fewer defences (in psychological terms) and the personality is vulnerable from without. Intervention can be effective which is quite impossible at other times.

I speak of the whole personality – not just of the cluster of ideas or feelings involved in the actual events of crisis.

However, there is a very special responsibility about our intervention in a crisis – intervention *must* be restricted to relevant matters. It is possible to convert or unconvert a person much more easily during crisis resolution because the general defences of the personality are low. It is not accidental that 'brain washing' techniques have as their basis the artificial production of crises.

We have a special responsibility not to impose our brand of political, religious, psychiatric or sociological dogmatism on our clients when they come to us for quite other reasons.

To return to *crisis resolution* – there seem to be *three phases* involved in the resolution of crisis:

1. Physical and mental *turmoil*
   Aimless activity or immobilisation
   Disorganisation of some degree – often great

2. *Painful preoccupation* with the past
   In psychiatric terms the person may *regress* to infantile or childhood methods of dealing with the world and with oneself. These methods include dependency, alcoholism, depression or withdrawal. If he finds these old methods either not workable in terms of a solution, or not acceptable in terms of his self-esteem, he may then go on to the third phase.

3. *Remobilisation*, activity, adjustment
   To simplify:
   Pain, digestion, action or
   shock, grief, action

It appears to be established that missing any of these phases leads to non-resolution, i.e. injury on a more or less permanent scale.

Problems are less painful than crises; they involve no disorganisation. No new solution (in terms of the personality) has to be found – it is merely a matter of sorting out already acquired functions and selecting an appropriate one.

Crisis presents pain and disorganisation and its resolution demands a change in the view of, or a readaptation to, the world, or the person – or both.

We have to allow clients *time* to get through the phases. Aid can only be effective in the second or third phase. We may need to protect the client during phase one.

Ego growth (increase in 'self-ness') can only occur during crisis resolution. A crisis successfully met leaves the person larger, more efficient, more capable than before – and permanently so. This underlies the necessity for the *solution to be found by the client*, not by the counsellor. If we ignore this: 1. We deny the client the possibility of growth. 2. We court dependency – non-resolution and regression to 'Daddy make it better'. It also explains why only *listening* is necessary on so many occasions, and why Samaritan volunteers are so valuable in this work.

There seems to be a sharp division between those with qualifications and those without. Do we use the committed volunteer, the human being who really cares about doing something for others, enough? Talking about pain or worry to someone truly sympathetic cuts tensions and distress to a manageable level. Once you've been able to talk to someone who's listened – really listened, for one of the great things in life is to listen, properly, and have time for others – it's of extraordinary benefit.

H.R.H. THE PRINCE OF WALES, in *The Standard*, 10–7–84

Depression – CHARLES BAGG*

Depression is a many headed monster. We shall consider two of the forms in which it occurs.

Endogenous depression

The first depressive syndrome (i.e. collection of symptoms) that I will mention is ENDOGENOUS DEPRESSION. 'Endogenous' means generated from within, not as a result of external misfortune.

The practical implication of this is that if you have got somebody with an endogenous depression, *don't think that you are going to make it better by tinkering about with the environment*, or *even by befriending them, except as the most effective means of getting them to the doctor*. It is a condition which is not primarily and predominantly due to external factors, and it is not going to be remedied by external factors. If you fail to recognise that, and try to do your stuff on behalf of the patient, sooner or later you are going to put your foot in it, and there may be a very tragic outcome. This I have seen happen, not with Samaritans but in other circumstances.

The answer, when you have diagnosed an endogenous depression, is to get it off your hands. Now by that I don't mean jettison the patient in an unkind way, but seek professional advice, and don't try to cope with the situation yourself. If you do and thereby fail to ameliorate the condition, the patient may commit suicide. Not everyone with endogenous depression will commit suicide – most of them don't, but it is a condition in which suicide is a known risk.

There are other unfortunate sequels – there will be a great

* From a talk given at The Samaritan's National Conference 1969.

deal of unhappiness that the individual will suffer, quite unnecessarily, because this condition is eminently curable. The unhappiness will be both for the individual patient and for the family. There will often be misunderstanding by the family, and when the family finally recognise with hindsight that the condition was in fact an illness, they will reproach themselves accordingly.

Loss of employment is another risk. The incompetence that this illness creates in individuals is liable to give them a reputation that they may not be able to live down, even after recovery, and they may, in fact, lose their jobs. Another thing that tends to happen is *marital disturbance*, and even, occasionally, a marital break-up. The depressed patient becomes very unattractive, and the marital partner, not understanding the reality of the situation, may construe the change as a loss of affection, and may go and seek affection elsewhere. For all these reasons it is important that this condition is diagnosed in the very *early stages*.

Usually when a patient comes to a GP, and still more to a psychiatrist, things have gone manifestly awry. Before that stage has arrived, any of these circumstances that I have just named may have developed, including suicide. *They may commit suicide before they ever get to the doctor.* Furthermore, anybody except a half-wit can diagnose endogenous depression in its advanced stages, in its clear cut form. To spot it in its incipient stages is a very different matter, and this is just the point at which you are likely to come in.

Endogenous depression comes on for no apparent reason, or if there is an alleged reason, that reason is in fact more apparent than real. Sometimes I must admit, this illness does seem to have been genuinely precipitated by some factor, but this factor is only something that has just been the last straw, it is not the essence of the condition.

The symptoms of this condition are, first a *decline in interest and initiative and emotional response*. Matters which had previously been of interest to the patient cease to form the centre of his attention. Work or domestic duties are liable to tail off. A degree of incompetence, which may not be recognised as pathological at that stage, begins to assert itself. The patient begins to spoil his daily work, not necessarily very grossly, but to people who are working closely with him it becomes apparent. Often people cover up for him, because he is usually a very nice person who has always been very conscientious.

Since this illness tends on the whole to come on the basis of a conscientious personality, the sufferer tends, with commendable stoicism, to struggle against the illness. In the early stages he often succeeds, and this obscures from the bystanders the fact that there is an illness at all. The patient will feel different, he will feel this coming on, but you may not notice it very much.

Another feature is *indecisiveness*. The person who previously had been at least capable of taking firm decisions – though he often tends to have been the sort of personality that rather laboriously weighs the pros and cons – will become indecisive. This, of course, is a thing that often gets under the skin of people working with him, and gets under the skin of the marital partner; and to the misfortune of his illness is added the misfortune of recriminations.

All these things are part and parcel of 'Psychomotor retardation' – which is exactly what it says – slowing up of the psychological processes and movement. In the extreme stage of this condition I have seen people so frozen that they have been brought into hospital on a stretcher in a condition that is known as depressive stupor – they just can't move. It is seldom that one gets to that stage, but in a moderately severe case they often present a picture rather like a film in slow motion – with droopy stance, depressive facial expression, and slowing of mental functions. This is very distressing to them, and they find that they have to make a conscious intentional effort to drag out of themselves thoughts which, before they became ill, would arise perfectly spontaneously. Their concentration tails off, they will tell you that they read the paper and at the end of it they don't know a word of what is in it. As the condition gathers momentum, they can no longer overcome the disabling influence of these symptoms and they are laid low by the illness; at that point they go to the doctor – if they haven't committed suicide before.

All these symptoms, characteristic of the early stages of the illness, may very well occur without the patient spontaneously informing you of the facts. He is not the sort of person, normally, and still less when he is ill, who wears his heart on his sleeve, and he just won't tell you these things. So *ask him* whether he is getting indecisive, ask him whether he is losing interest; if once you suspect the diagnosis don't just leave him to tell you, because he may very well not do so, and you will have missed the significance of the whole thing.

There are certain qualities of thought which are extremely characteristic of this condition and the cardinal feature, I would say, is *self-reproach*. He will blame himself, quite irrationally, for things which superficially might have a basis in reason, but which in fact are rooted in illness. This is where your skill in distinguishing between the two has to come into play – he will accuse himself irrationally of things, and in the gross degree of the illness the patient will say something which is so clearly delusional that nobody could possibly fail to recognise that he is in fact ill.

A delusion by definition is a false belief that is not amenable to reason. It is not founded in logic and it can't be dispelled by logic. So that if you try to use a logical approach, which would seem on the face of it the sensible thing to do, you are going to do no good at all, you are going to make things worse. Another delusion that is common in greater or lesser degree in this condition, is the *delusion of futility*. He feels, in the extreme anyway, that everything is utterly black, there is no hope, there is no salvation. Again, if you don't recognise the essentially morbid origin of this, you are liable to try to talk him out of it.

There may be delusions of *hypochondriasis* – that is to say, believing that there is bodily disease when in fact none exists. Such delusions are very characteristic of the depression of middle life and the senile period. They are very characteristic indeed of the menopausal depression, the involutional depressions (what used to be termed involutional melancholia), which occur in middle-aged women at the change of life.

Involutional melancholia is characterised typically by very bizarre hypochondriacal delusions, for example, a lady with agitated depression, who believed that her gullet stopped 'here' – I don't know what she thought happened to the food after that. This was one of the hypochondriacal delusions of involutional melancholia.

A further example, particularly characteristic in the senile period, is delusions of *poverty*. One has seen people, who are unquestionably well off who believe absolutely that they are financially ruined.

Loss of appetite is another very characteristic depressive symptom. They go off their food, or, even if they don't actually reduce the intake, they don't enjoy their food as they did. So this condition, anorexia, is very characteristic indeed of depressive illness.

Associated with this is loss of *sexual appetite*, loss of sexual interest, sexual capacity, sexual enjoyment, and of course this symptom tends, as you can imagine, to feed into the depressive tendency to self-reproach. They tend to feel that they are letting their marital partners down, and the marital partner may in fact feel rejected.

One more symptom that you really need to commit to memory is *insomnia*. This doesn't mean that because we sleep badly we have got depression, but there is a certain pattern to this insomnia which is characteristic of depressives. They wake during the small hours of the morning, only to be tormented with this ceaseless round of delusionally coloured unconstructive ruminations, as a result of which in the small hours of the morning they may get up and go downstairs and 'take a bottle', and that's the end of that.

Diurnal variation means that they are typically worse first thing in the morning. As the day goes on the condition improves.

There are certain phases in which *suicide* is a particularly high risk. Paradoxically, it is not so much when they are utterly immobilised by depression that the risk is highest, but when they are *going into the depression* – that is when you may come into it – and when they are *coming out of it*. When the depression is maximal, they are so retarded as to be incapable of the initiative, mental and physical, to make a suicide attempt. But give them three or four electric treatments, for example, and they are comparatively better, but they are still deluded and wretched; they are capable by then of taking the suicidal action, and this is the time when it is likely to happen. Also, when they are first going into the depression, particularly if they are receiving any form of anti-depressant treatment as out-patients, and are not under immediate observation in hospital – this is the time when you need to be particularly vigilant.

One feature of unmixed depression is that it can be satisfactorily cured, dispelled. I still never cease to wonder at the metamorphosis that one produces over three or four weeks or less in these cases. It is a condition, most often, from which they completely recover. The immediate outlook is very good, and there is no residual defect, but it is an illness which tends to recur. (So if you know of anyone who has had such an attack, just keep on the look-out for recurrence, and nip it in the bud.)

The person who becomes depressed is often an *obsessive personality*. Many of us are normally obsessive about details, about order, about tidiness, but an obsessional personality may develop a psychosis in which the person loses touch with reality and suffers from delusions – he does not understand that he is ill, but believes that he is guilty, useless or unclean.

Features of endogenous depression

These are psychomotor retardation, indecisiveness, self-reproach, the sense of futility, hypochondriasis, delusions of poverty, loss of appetites, the pattern of insomnia, diurnal variation; and the dangerous phases, going into the depression and partial recovery.

Reactive depression

By contrast, reactive depression is explicable and comprehensible in terms of the circumstances that preceded its onset. That is to say, if someone suddenly loses all their stocks and shares, they may go into a reactive depression. The condition subsides when these precipitating circumstances are resolved.

If, on the other hand, it so happened that an endogenous depression followed, perhaps precipitated by a financial disaster, it would not make one scrap of difference if I won all the football pools.

So you can spot the reactive depression, partly by a process of exclusion. You don't typically find it preceded by an obsessional personality, you don't find the diurnal variation, you don't find many of the other symptoms of endogenous depression; and they are not concerned primarily and predominantly and fundamentally with self-reproach, futility, hypochondriasis, etc. – they are preoccupied with whatever misfortune brought on this state. They are not typically retarded in the way that the endogenous depressive is. Indeed, if you have a co-existing element of hysteria in the condition, as you fairly frequently do, you will find that there is a flamboyant display of grief quite often.

There is no denying that they are depressed, but it is a different quality, it has a different essential origin, different management, and a different outcome.

The content of the reactive depression does not spread into the irrational ideas which characterise the endogenous depressive. In the reactive depression, when once you are satisfied that this is what you are dealing with, don't be afraid of helping them in their crisis, by befriending plus, if necessary, referral.

After-treatment for depression – W. Linford Rees

Severe depression is treatable with drugs. There are ways, however, in which Samaritans can help the sufferer. They can befriend, show interest, and give support. This is helpful in all types of depression, but in severe cases may not produce much in the way of improvement. Nevertheless it is important and appreciated by the patient.

For the patient who has undergone treatment and is discharged home, it is often a critical time when commonsense and enlightened help with the patient and with his relations is so important. One has to try and live in the boots of one and the shoes of the other. Consider the patient first – he may still have some residue of his illness, he may have some feelings of inferiority and alienation as a result of his hospitalisation. He may have practical problems with re-employment. Consider the family, with their complex attitudes towards the patient's recent illness – there is bound to be some apprehensiveness and concern for his future, some exasperation, perhaps, with any residual symptoms. Befriending by Samaritans can provide invaluable help in one of the most distressing and incapacitating illnesses which afflict mankind.

The incurable case – P. W. W. Leach

As in other fields of medicine, psychiatry is still frequently faced with the incurable and untreatable problem. Depression is no exception in this field. There are some forms even of endogenous depression that do not fully recover after the most skilful and generous use of physical methods. This may be because of an underlying and insidious organic change such as cerebral arteriosclerosis, or it may be because of an admixture of some other mental disorder such as schizophrenia or hysteria, or it may be some as yet undiscovered biochemical abnormality. And then again with the reactive and neurotic forms of depression one must accept that there *are* insoluble practical problems in life which even the most devoted doctors or social workers are unable to ameliorate. The aim must then be to support the patient with the shared knowledge of their difficulties, as is achieved by Samaritan befriending. It cannot be pretended that the depression is being alleviated but the life of the sufferer is being made more supportable.

'Masked' depression – William Sargant

Why is it that so many people, having consulted their general practitioners and even psychiatrists, almost straight away go off and still kill themselves? The answer, or a very large part of it, lies in the existence of large numbers of states of *'masked' depression*, which need special psychological training and skills to recognise. Doctors, whatever their philosophical viewpoint, do not in practice stand aside and let patients kill themselves, if it can be avoided. Yet thousands and thousands do either attempt or succeed in doing so each year, often with the very drugs prescribed by their doctor.

Let us get down to the basics of this problem. Around one-third of the patients coming to St Thomas's, for instance, for various tests, X-rays and other physical examinations, are people of often sterling worth, who have worked regularly, supported families and relatives, helped others and been, in all respects, model citizens. Then gradually, or suddenly, they start to feel a variety of pains, sometimes in the head, or in the back of the neck. They may also complain of dryness of the mouth and throat. Their chest or heart may pain them periodically, or their stomach starts to get a vague tense and uneasy feeling. Constipation can be a major worry, or faulty eyesight, not helped by glasses.

Along with the development of these physical symptoms and abnormal feelings, they may start to experience intolerable anxiety for no known reason. Perhaps they have been through a period of stress which is now passing. They also start to become very tired for no known reason, or they may start waking early and regularly for the first time in their life. Some alternatively sleep deeply all night and still feel just as abnormally tired the following day, when they try to do their normal work. For many, jobs that were easy for them for years start to become difficult. Making decisions over simple matters also worries them. They become more irritable with people they really love, and later they may start to blame themselves for the most foolish things, and search their past lives for causes for self-blame.

When asked whether, in fact, they are depressed, they will generally say they are more tense and anxious. And they almost invariably attribute their increased anxiety to the recent onset of the physical symptoms, of which they are now complaining, and what these symptoms may portend, such as brain tumour, stomach cancers, coronary heart disease and the like. And it is then, to find out about these symptoms in somebody usually so well, that the patient is sent for special tests to a teaching hospital or elsewhere.

It is now that a mistake can be made by general practitioners, physicians and psychiatrists alike. This is to examine the patient very carefully, perhaps do all sorts of tests and X-rays and then tell him that he is normal and there is nothing very much the matter with him. Perhaps, even worse, is to say it is 'all nerves', which means nothing serious to too many doctors and patients, and to simply prescribe sedatives.

What is such a man or woman then to do?

They begin to think the only thing they can do, as they become more and more incapacitated and yet supposedly medically quite well, is to put themselves out of the way, to stop, by committing suicide, being a 'medically well' total burden to their family and themselves. How many patients, with a missed depressive illness, have gone to their death with their doctor's supposedly heartening reassurance in their ears, that there is nothing the matter with them that a bit of will-power won't put right?

Clinical treatment of depression – William Sargant

1. *Drug treatment*

In recent years, psychiatry and general medicine have become equipped with two groups of powerful and effective drugs, almost specific in certain states of depression and anxiety. If general practitioners could learn their skilled use and not be too worried by side effects that happen with all powerful and effective drugs in medicine as a whole, they could themselves cope with around 75% of the anxiety states and depressions in persons of adequate personality, without any need to refer them for specialised psychotherapy and psychiatric treatment. Several practitioners have already found this out, having taken the trouble to learn about them.

Drug manufacturers tend to claim that their particular anti-depressant drug covers the whole group of depressed patients, and muddle doctors up a lot with their excessive claims. There is a tendency to rush from one new anti-depressant to the next new one, although they may be the same group of drugs under different trade names. The two main groups of drugs must be discussed since too many people think they overlap where a few patients made worse by one are made better by the other and vice versa. The MAOIs (Mono-amine Oxidase Inhibitor drugs) are extremely valuable in states of anxiety and reactive depression in patients, who may have been ill for years, but are still fighting their symptoms. They are particularly valuable in phobic anxiety states, where people get panicky at going into the street, attending church or the cinema, and going in trains, etc. These people are also depressed and can be suicidal in their despair about their restricted life. The MAOIs are also valuable in fatigue states, where people sleep deeply all night, and wake up just as tired in the morning, as opposed to those who wake up early in an extremely agitated state. Unfortunately, the MAOIs require certain dietary restrictions, and severe headaches when the wrong foodstuffs are taken frighten some doctors and patients off them. Nevertheless, unless they are fully used in states of depression, large numbers of people will remain ill, and possibly suicidal, since the MAOI responding depressions and anxiety states do badly with the other group of anti-depressants called the *tricyclics*. These are much more useful in patients who are retarded and slow with early waking and guilt. In fact, the 'masked' depressions often do best with the MAOIs, and the obvious melancholias with the tricyclics. And there are other neurotic depressions, which do best of all when both groups are combined. This is now quite safe if certain precautions are taken.

People have such silly attitudes to mental illness and drugs. Few would think it wrong to take insulin for diabetes or Vit. B12 for pernicious anaemia – both killing diseases. Yet some baulk at using drugs in depressive illnesses, which can be just as lethal, judging by the approximately 200,000 suicidal attempts each year. One of the important things about the anti-depressants is that there is no need to increase the dose despite years on them. And please do not encourage patients to try to 'get down to the root' of their problems, when they are depressed. Lots of depressive illnesses are inherited, run in families, occur for no known reason, and respond to drugs: we do not yet know why. Such a position is common in medicine, where we do not know even how aspirin works. *Psychological probing can be very dangerous in depression*. Wait until the patient is much better with drugs or other treatment, and then see if he can be further helped psychotherapeutically without risk of precipitating a suicide attempt by trying to uncover material the patient just cannot cope with. ECT is a much older treatment than the new drugs. But there are still many suicidal depressives who will quickly get well with it, even when the drugs have failed to help.

2. *Electrical treatment – P. W. W. Leach*

Still sometimes used in *endogenous depression* is *electroplexy* (electrical treatment). This entails the passage of a measured amount of current for a measured time through the frontal region of the brain while the patient is asleep with short-acting anaesthetic and muscle-relaxants given by the vein. One treatment lasts about three minutes and the patient is awake and up and about again in half an hour. Out-patients are able to return home and resume work on the same morning. About six treatments given twice weekly are sufficient. There are no ill-effects other than muzziness or headache for a period after each treatment and minor disturbances of memory lasting for a few weeks after a course of treatment.

Causes of psychiatric disorder – Kenneth Rawnsley

Psychiatric disorder is not uniformly distributed throughout the population. It occurs in pockets. It occurs in certain sections of society more than in others. It appears to be more prevalent in some conditions in women than in men. It is certainly more frequent in the elderly than it is in younger categories and it may be possible in time to throw some light on to problems of causation, because this is a field where we are at the present time sorely in need of information. We know a certain amount about the cause of mental disorder. We know also how very ignorant we are on this matter. And we have to use all kinds of methods to forward this aim of discovering the causes of psychiatric illness: the clinical method, the bedside method, methods derived from the basic sciences, chemistry, physics, physiology and so on. The epidemiological method is one of these tools which we have and which we can use for this purpose, because if we can find certain sections of society, certain kinds of people, groups of people who have high rates for specific mental disorders and, conversely, if we find people who have low rates for these conditions, we may be able to derive clues about the causal factors operative. For example, it has been known for many years now that the prevalence of the psychiatric disorder schizophrenia, which is a serious condition, is highest in the unskilled section of society, what the Registrar-General calls 'Social Class V' – far higher in the members of Social Class V than it is among other social categories of the population. At first it was thought that this might indicate that something about the way of life in Social Class V was productive of schizophrenia. We now know that it is more likely that the high prevalence of schizophrenia in Social Class V is a consequence of the disease rather than a cause, because if you develop schizophrenia you may become socially less competent, you may lose your job, which may be a skilled job, and you may slide down the social scale. By the time you enter a psychiatric hospital, or by the time you become a declared case as it were, your social position may be that of an unskilled worker and therefore this produces an apparently high prevalence in Social Class V. This is an example of the difficulties which the method presents, the problems of interpretation which one has to cope with in using this method, and there are many such problems to be met and sorted out before we can really gain the maximum use from this method of enquiry.

Social pressures towards suicide – Ivor Mills

Everyone must pay homage to the new god which is called *efficiency*. More money must be earned by more work until everyone is pushed to the very limit of his tolerance . . .

Workers pushed to the limit of their tolerance no longer conform to the principles of economic theory; they are no longer reasonable. When they strike, they are not crying for help: they are telling you that the conditions of life are intolerable. From animal studies we know that when the breakdown of social order begins it may progress with fantastic speed. We are witnessing today the early stages of the breakdown of civilisation in the most highly developed countries. It is the result of too many people and too great a drive to reach too much affluence, in short, too much competition. If life is to be made more tolerable we must have a dramatic reduction in the population: we must reduce considerably the competition in schools, colleges and universities: we must include some degree of inefficiency in every job carried out by a man or woman: we must be content with less affluence.

Potential suicides – George Day

Most suicide risks are among ordinary people with no mental illness – ordinary, everyday people stricken with worry, dispirited by disaster, beaten down by their personal problems. To enumerate some of the misfortunes that can dispirit us: bereavement, loss of security, loss of job, redundancy, loss of social status; the failures: matrimonial failure, failure to get expected promotion, failure to pass examinations; and the *fear* of failure, because the students take their overdoses *before* the exams which they dread, not usually after them. Nagging anxieties that can't be relieved, about one's health, about the health of one's loved ones, and – loneliness.

These life situations are situations in which the victim may feel a bit shamefaced, a bit to blame, so he doesn't want to advertise them to anyone he knows, certainly not to his family, nor to his doctor, nor his priest. He's bursting to get it off his chest, discuss it with somebody. But it must be somebody he doesn't know, whose confidentiality he can trust, and whom he need never see again if and when he gets through his trouble.

The majority of suicides are not mentally ill – Richard Fox

Assessment of the suicidal episode requires careful consideration of the act itself and of the life situation in which the act took place: of the state of affairs to which the suicidal episode appeared, at that time, to be the answer. Usually the wrong answer. Many would say that it is always the wrong answer though one does from time to time find situations in which one has to admit that in all logic suicide just does make sense and in which one might oneself very well choose suicide; underlining a point which is often forgotten, that not every suicidal person is mentally ill. It is easy to assume that anyone who feels like ending it all must be *ipso facto* insane, but this is an immature view, reflecting personal anxieties about death, and not one which fits the facts. Clear evidence of psychotic disorder is only found in about one-third of cases of successful suicide, and of less significant mental instability in a further one-third, though these figures are often disputed.

Oh, the comfort, the inexpressible comfort, of feeling safe with a person; having neither to weigh thoughts nor measure words, but to pour them all out just as they are, chaff and grain together, knowing that a faithful hand will take and sift them, keep what is worth keeping, and then, with the breath of kindness, blow the rest away.

GEORGE ELIOT

Assessing suicide risk – ROY VINING

The Samaritans' response to a suicidal caller must be proportionate to his danger, so careful enquiry into his suicidal feelings and intentions is essential if fatal errors are to be avoided.

The caller may mention suicidal feelings himself, or hint at them – 'I can't go on', 'I wish I was out of this mess', 'No way out' or the like: hints need to be followed up at once by asking the client what he means, lest he feel the subject is taboo. If he provides no such opening, then the Samaritan must ask, either gradually – 'Do you feel life isn't worth living?' – 'Have you ever felt like ending it all?' or straight out: 'Have you turned to The Samaritans because you feel suicidal?'

If the caller does feel suicidal, there are three essentials to be found out:

1. Is there a *suicide plan*? If so, what is it, when, and perhaps where?
2. Are the *means* available?
3. Has any *previous* suicidal act been made, or started? If so, what, and when? To what extent did the caller intend to die?

These form a quite natural sequence and need not seem like a questionnaire.

The suicide plan

The suicide plan and its intended timing are the main indicators of the immediate risk. Alongside the plan and any history of previous suicidal acts, the caller's story may have revealed other risk factors which should be taken into account: if a person is old, ill, addicted, depressive, isolated or rejected, or devoid of hope, these things (listed here in order of growing importance) will increase the risk – they are the things which place the caller 'in a high risk group'.

Lethality scoring

Lethality scoring offers a convenient summary of what we need to know, and by assigning numerical weightings to the risk factors provides a rough measure of a client's danger in a form that is easy to use and remember. Many Branches are using it in their instruction of new volunteers.

LETHALITY SCORING TABLE

Start on left by scoring the Suicide Plan (chief indicator of immediate risk), then add points for anything relevant on the right (mostly long-term factors).

SUICIDE RISK	**Score	OTHER FACTORS	Add to score
Imminent sudden death	8	Previous suicidal acts up to	4
Imminent slow method suicide	7	Absence of hope; loss of faith	3*
Planning sudden death	6	Recent broken relationship	3
Planning slow method suicide	5	Isolation: Rejection	3*
Planning a suicide gamble	4	Depressive illness (endogenous)	2
Planning a suicide gesture	3	Dependence on alcohol or drugs	2
Definite suicidal thoughts, no plan	2	Possession of means of suicide	2
Toying vaguely with idea of suicide	1	Putting affairs in order	2
No suicidal thoughts	0	Over 60; Male; Ill; Chronic pain	1*

**Score one figure from this side. *Score everything that applies.

ASK ABOUT SUICIDE RISK IN *EVERY* CASE AND AT *EVERY* CONTACT!

Examples

1. A widower aged sixty-seven with painful arthritis, living alone in a twelfth floor flat, who took an overdose last year (intending to die and prevented by an unexpected visitor), has made a new will and intends to jump from his balcony. For planning sudden death he scores 6 (8 if he means to do it immediately). Then add 4 for his previous overdose, 3 for his hopelessness, 3 for his isolation, 2 for the twelfth floor (he has the means for his plan), 2 for the new will (putting his affairs in order), plus 1 for age *and* 1 because he's male *and* 1 for his pain. So he scores 23 or 25, and we'll try not to let him out of our sight till he feels differently.
2. A girl who openly took eight aspirins during a row with

her boy friend and threatens to do it again unless he sees her more often, scores 3 for planning a suicide gesture, plus 0 or 1 for the previous gesture. Having heard her out fully we could let her go.

Study of such examples, and intermediate ones, suggests that a lethality score of over 20 requires that we stay with the caller till the risk declines. 14 or over requires us to arrange another contact less urgently; below that it's probably fair enough to invite the caller to contact us again if he/she wishes (unless there are separate reasons for keeping in positive touch).

The relation of response to risk can be summarised thus:

LETHALITY SCORE	LEVEL OF RISK	LEVEL OF RESPONSE
	Attempt in progress	Arrange treatment if caller willing
7 or 8 on left or total of 20+	On the brink	Stay with caller
14 to 19	High risk	*Fix* another contact *very* soon
6 to 13	Moderate risk	*Fix* another contact
1 to 5	Slight risk	Hear client out and let go (unless
0 on the left	No suicidal thoughts	other reasons for further contact)

When lethality scoring was first introduced at a Leaders' School at Swanwick, Derbyshire, some anxiety was expressed that the spontaneity of the 'befriending response' of the Samaritan volunteer might be impaired by attention to lethality calculations. This must certainly be avoided by so familiarising the applicants in the Preparation Classes with the procedure that it becomes second nature. The most relaxed possible conversation with a caller seriously at risk should in any case provide information which will enable a Director or Leader to score his/her lethality.

Keep on asking

Since suicide risk fluctuates we must never fall into the trap of regarding our original assessment as permanently valid (whether expressed as a number or not). On the contrary, we must be alert for changes – especially upswings that can result in death; and this means that we must *keep on asking*, and make a fresh assessment at every encounter.

One further warning: failure to find out everything relevant will result in too low a score and a false sense of security. This is not a fault of the lethality scoring system – it is a fact of life that however lethality is assessed, if it isn't done properly the danger will be underestimated and clients put at risk.

Summary

Never ignore possible suicide hints.

Assess the risk by asking in detail about suicidal feelings, *every* time.

Match The Samaritans' response to the client's danger.

All of us on this beautiful earth are terminal; no one is getting out of here alive.

DR IRENE KASSORLA, *Nice Girls Do*

Danger signs of acute suicide risk

1. Client withdrawn, cannot relate to you. Medical aid needed.
2. Family history of suicide.
3. Earlier attempts at suicide.
4. Definite idea of how suicide would be committed. The tidying up of affairs indicates suicide is being planned.
5. Anxious tone to depressive picture.
6. Dependence on alcohol or drugs.
7. Some painful physical illness and long sleep disturbance.
8. Feeling of uselessness. In elderly, lack of acceptance of retirement.
9. Isolation, loneliness and uprooting.
10. The possibility of having to live with few human contacts.
11. Lack of a philosophy of life such as a comforting type of religious faith.
12. Financial worries.
13. Within the period of the rise and fall in mood, the most dangerous time is often when the client appears better. Now he has enough energy to kill himself.

After the suicide question – ALBERT JEWELL

Before becoming Chairman it was my privilege for four years to serve as Vice-Chairman of The Samaritans with responsibility for training in the movement. Realising what an enormous task this is, one of the things I got round to doing was to call together a 'think-tank' to take an overview of what we do in this vital area. I had some pretty clear expectations of what the agenda should be, but in the event the think-tank threw them all out, and said, quite rightly, that we must address ourselves to a much more radical task. What we must do, they urged, is to ask what is the purpose of The Samaritans, and how well do we fulfil that purpose. Because, once selected, all training must fit us to carry out our work more effectively, for the sake of our callers. They went on to answer their own questions. We *say* that we're here to befriend the suicidal and despairing, but by and large (they maintained) we don't do it awfully well.

It is not difficult to find supporting evidence for this diagnosis. Some of it comes from outside The Samaritans; for example, we know that the suicide rate in the UK has been gradually creeping up a little over recent years, after the large and steady decrease from 1963, despite the near-saturation of the country by Samaritan Branches. And research projects on over-dosers who survive consistently show that almost none even thought to contact The Samaritans, not that parasuicides could be expected to. And there is a lot more evidence from our own statistics and experience. We know, for example, that we do not seem to be reaching the highest risk group at all, that of older men. Very many of our calls are of a one-off nature and of very short duration, so we cannot reckon to have gone very deep with the majority of our callers. Probably the suicide boxes on our report sheets get filled up in less than 50% of cases. And it has to be admitted that in busy Branches the lines are often clogged with chronic callers whom we are probably not really helping, so that those in crisis can actually be prevented from getting through at their moment of utter desperation. The conclusion from this disquieting evidence would seem to be that the suicidal are simply not coming to us in any great numbers (which would be a very serious indictment, if true) or, worse still, that they are, but we fail to recognise them or we do not actually help them.

Now, obviously the picture is not as uniformly black as that or we would have packed up a long time ago. We have indeed learned a lot from the factors I have mentioned and have responded to them in various ways, for example, adopting a slightly higher profile as an organisation, reaching out more to the suicidal, encouraging the taking of third-party referrals and the offering of follow-up, and especially in improving our selection and training. This has been most marked in recent years in two directions:

1. First, emphasising *the asking of the suicide question.* It is amazing that after more than thirty years we still need to convince volunteers that this is what we are here for, and that we all still try to wriggle out of it by one means or another – often by maintaining that we did not think it really relevant to *that* particular caller, e.g. 'it was only old George' or 'it was quite obvious that all she wanted was . . .' But we are getting better at it, or so the report sheets glimpsed during Branch visits would seem to indicate.

It seems to me that our difficulties in this area are threefold:

(i) We are still not totally convinced that asking the question will not put the idea of suicide into the minds of our callers. *This* is, of course, a hardy annual at any Samaritan gathering, and reflects a very worthy fear were it to have any grounds in reality. Psychiatrists and suicidologists are unanimous in saying that it is just not possible to put the idea into another person's mind in that sort of way (they will simply brush it aside), but that it is a wonderful safety valve and therapy to be given permission to say YES to the suicide question and the opportunity to pour out some of the dark and shameful feelings that have been dammed up. We need to keep reminding ourselves of this.

(ii) We don't know *how* to ask the question, so we end up evading it or botching the issue. And it does need a great deal of sensitivity to judge the right moment and the right manner in which to introduce the question. My suggestion is that we listen to other Samaritans and see how they do it and so find some way that is natural to us, and be prepared to tailor it gently to the needs of any particular caller. Personally I usually find it best to be pretty explicit, whilst trying not to sound as if the caller's feelings are reprehensible in any way, e.g. 'Things do sound pretty bad – do they seem so bad that you've felt like ending it all?' The main thing is to be brave enough to ask it in our own way, and not to get thrown by a brush-off or to be misled by appearances (e.g. the 'laughing suicide'); we may need to go back to the question again to get a more honest answer. And remember – even if the report sheets show that the caller was not suicidal last time, or has never been suicidal, that does not mean that he is not suicidal this time. So it is always right to ask.

I seem to remember from my dim and distant school days that there are two ways of asking a question in Latin: the little word *nonne* inviting an affirmative reply, and the little word *num* expecting the negative. I cannot help thinking that we all too often ask the suicide question hoping for a 'no' and fearful of a 'yes', and that this fear communicates itself to our callers who recognise the signal and draw back to protect us from something they sense we may be unable to bear.

(iii) But part of the difficulty also undoubtedly lies in our making the suicide question a stopping point (to get it over with, with some relief, and fill in the report sheets accordingly) rather than as a starting point because we tend not to know where to go from there.

2. And it is here where the second great improvement in our preparation and practice in recent years comes in – the use of *lethality scoring* on the front of the case sheets for the first

contact and as a continuing column on all subsequent sheets. Lethality scoring is based upon certain definite criteria that we can apply, which are broadly speaking as follows:

(i) Has the caller the plan and the means for self-destruction, ranging from vague thoughts at the bottom of the scale, through slow death by tablets where there is perhaps an even chance of being discovered in time, to sudden death, e.g. by shotgun from which there can be no chance of escape once it has been initiated?

(ii) Has the caller a *history* of such attempts, for he is probably at much greater risk if he has?

(iii) Are there suggestive *background factors* present that make the situation worse and suicide more likely? for example, is he elderly? has she suffered a broken relationship? is he living on his own? is she an alcoholic? etc.

These therefore are the sorts of consideration that can give us some indication of where to go beyond the suicide question when the answer is YES – these are the areas we can explore. And it is on this sort of basis that we are asked to rate the caller on a scale 0–9 and to do so not just once but at every subsequent contact. Such a rating can be an invaluable aid in alerting a leader or director to a worsening in a caller's situation. But to work effectively it does need to be applied consistently throughout the Branch. Too often, we find, this particular column is left blank. We need of course to remember that it can be only a rough indicator, never an absolute guide: someone seemingly of a low rating can catch us out by killing himself, and someone with a very high rating can go on surviving indefinitely. Again, callers will vary from occasion to occasion, which is why we must be prepared to ask the suicide question and explore the suicide and background factors at each and every contact.

Now, all that I have said so far about asking the suicide question and applying the lethality scale comes of good solid Samaritan experience and can help us from a factual point of view to fill up the report sheets effectively, but the trouble is that they may still not be very helpful to the caller, and may even become a substitute and let-out for really allowing them to pour out their black feelings and plumb the depths of their despair. Which is why, to go back to where we started, my think-tank homed in on this particular area and declared that, by and large, we do not deliver the goods as we ought because we do not adequately explore the suicidal feelings of our callers. We hold back from the abyss. Well, I must admit that my initial reaction was one of scepticism, if not of rank disbelief, when I considered all the wonderful Samaritans I knew who surely did deliver the goods – and I did not think it was true of me either! Hence my determination to put it to the test the very next time I picked up the phone on duty. The outcome was an ineffective role-play which left me needing to be scraped up off the floor by my leader who luckily happened to be right there!

The trouble is, as I discovered on that traumatic duty, that steering into suicidal feelings rather than away from them, choosing to go over and down some way into the abyss with our callers, is so against all our natural inclinations that we need all the time to go on recalling ourselves to the task. It is a terribly difficult thing to do. Surely it cannot be coincidental that whenever I have made a sustained effort to steer into suicide, some quite remarkable things have come out; whenever I have neglected to do so or felt too drained to go very far in that direction, things have stayed very much on the surface.

But *why* do we find it so difficult? This was the question to which the think-tank then addressed itself, now that its Chairman was a late convert to the cause! The answer, we think, is quite simple to state but hard to do anything about – it is mostly sheer *fear*: the fear of the unknown and of darkness, and especially the dread of death, which is uncharted and terrifying territory. So, when the abyss looms up with a caller, our automatic reaction and natural instinct is to draw back from it, or to find some way of going round it – even to jump over it – anything rather than consenting to go down into it just as far as our caller wants and needs. This fear is a complex one and would appear to operate at both conscious and unconscious levels:

(i) The conscious level is, I suppose, the level at which we might be prepared to justify ourselves with our fellow-Samaritans, e.g. by contending that the vast majority of our callers are *not* in fact suicidal, therefore to go totally overboard on this tack would be to frighten them all away; or by thinking that if we allow them to over-indulge their misery and wallow in their despair, we may actually encourage the death-wish in them, whereas our job is surely to haul them up and out of the abyss, in other words to steer them *out* of suicide. This, I suppose, is a more sophisticated variant of the fear that talking about suicide with callers may plant the idea in their minds.

(ii) But it is probably the unconscious or less conscious levels of fear that are even more significant, two of which perhaps should be brought out into the open:

(a) First of all there is the very understandable fear of getting out of our depth, of encouraging our callers to let out all sorts of horrors which we are then totally unable to deal with, so that we may actually lose the caller, even in the ultimate sense. So, under this sort of pressure, we tend to resort sooner or later (and probably without realising it) to all those things our initial preparation warned us against and that the 'bad angel' in my role-play reintroduced: talking rather than listening to what is scarcely bearable; establishing facts rather than allowing feelings to be poured out; solving problems (all very non-directively, of course!) instead of soaking up the caller's sense of hopelessness – and we end up able to fill up the case sheets with some measurable results at least. Because the opposite is all but unbearable: to take it all deep down in our guts, to go down, down, down, into what we fear may be a bottomless pit, and to have the caller end up apparently still determined to end their life – all this is to end up feeling hopeless and helpless ourselves. It's all terribly draining and we know we cannot take too much of that kind of 'failure'. Yet we know also, paradoxically, that it is only out of such seeming 'failure' that any chance of Samaritan 'success' can come. For what our callers require of us is simply that we do what we say we are here to do: go on listening, go on befriending the despairing caller; in that we have the courage to go over the abyss holding their hand, and down as far as they wish, even to the very bottom, refusing to draw the line and back out somewhere on the way (though we will be sorely tempted to do so), because to do that some way down would certainly be to leave our callers in a far worse state than when they mustered enough courage to ring us. For what they are seeking is not a slick solution, nor someone to hoist them up prematurely, but simply a presence, another person, a companion to hold their hand and go with them (out of *both* our depths), and to reassure them they are not alone, that someone does care. In that companionship and caring there can be the beginnings upon which a new and more hopeful attitude may possibly begin to emerge and grow, terribly fragile though it is. So, although it is a terribly hard and demanding thing to do, we do not actually need tremendous specialist skills to steer into this dark and fearsome area: proper preparation certainly, a great deal of courage and sensitivity, yes, and above all a tremendous amount of support for one another. That way, we shall be able to go down with our caller without staying down, certainly without going under, and, at any rate, with the possibility that they will come up again with us.

(b) The other unconscious or scarcely conscious fear has to do not so much with our callers as with ourselves: the fear that if we enter into another person's suicidal feelings where is that going to leave us because we shall expose our own deepest dreads? Death, as we know, is (at any rate in our western society) such a taboo subject, such a mystery, such a dread, that our defences against it run both high and deep. But proper Samaritan befriending, whether we like it or not, is inevitably going to expose us to the pain of the bereavements we have suffered, the suicidal thoughts we may have entertained, and our own unresolved attitude to our own death, and all this can be too threatening to bear. So, going some way at least towards recognising and coming to terms with these issues ought really to figure rather more largely in our selection procedures and in our initial preparation and ongoing training. But one needs to sound a very real word of caution here: this is a very tricky and traumatic area in which to venture, and over-eager instructors need to beware. Perhaps we need to be humble enough to ask the help of others more skilled and experienced than ourselves, such as the branch Psychiatric consultant, if suitable, or an established bereavement counsellor. And of course we need to recognise that our own attitude to death is not something we shall be able to resolve once and for all. It is bound to evolve and change, so it will need constant personal re-assessment. All I would plead for is that we at least make a start in that direction.

In the end, I suppose it comes down to this. That we hold back for fear that if we go over and down into the abyss we may never come out again. But, for our suicidal callers, it is quite literally true that *unless* they find someone who will go that way with them they are certainly most unlikely to come up at all. And, when you think about it, who else but the Samaritans offer to do this? Who else but the Samaritans can be expected to do it? Let's do it! And let's help one another to do it.

To whom shall I speak today?
  I am laden with misery
  through lack of an intimate . . .
Death is in my sight today
  like the clearing of the sky,
  like a man attracted thereby to
  what he knows not.

Death is in my sight today,
  like the longing of a man to see home
  when he has spent many years held in captivity.

A dispute over suicide, Egypt, before 2000 BC, ANON

Befriending those who cannot cope – IVOR H. MILLS

People deliberately perform acts of self-injury and run the risk of killing themselves when the coping mechanism of the brain is completely exhausted. An understanding of how best to help them depends upon an appreciation of the means by which challenges to the coping mechanism may lead on to failure of this mechanism.

In the majority of cases they know that they are faced with problems with which they can no longer cope. So often they say 'I couldn't cope any more'. What they do is an effort to escape from the situation and if in escaping they risk death, they do not care. Almost always there is a final trigger which makes them perform the act, which in most cases is to take an overdose of drugs.

The most critical time to talk to them is just as they are recovering from the effect of drugs. At that time they are most ready to talk about what has happened. Sometimes, if they sense that there is not a receptive ear, they will refer only to the final trigger which initiated the act. Characteristically, they will have thought about taking the overdose for less than fifteen minutes before they did it. This final trigger is often something which appears too trivial to justify the risk of suicide. Here lies the clue to successful help for the person. If the trigger were accepted as the only challenge to the coping mechanism it would be impossible to understand, let alone help, the individual.

At the time when they are most ready to talk one can usually obtain the details of the repeated challenges in recent months – yes, months, not usually just days or weeks. If there have not been repeated episodes demanding exercise of the coping process in the brain, there will have been a longer term continuous, grumbling problem.

The arousal mechanism

Challenges to the brain represent problems to be solved, even if it is only to decide how to go on living with someone who is a continuous strain to live with. In trying to solve these problems the brain gets into a more excited state, i.e., the level of arousal is raised. It is then quicker and more efficient in solving single problems. If the challenges represent learning at school or doing mental work to earn one's living, the same elevation of arousal occurs. Major upsets in one's life may lead to sleep disturbance because the high arousal persists from one day to the next. Repeated major disturbances may lead to failure of the brain to cope with them and an underlying depression becomes manifest. Enjoyable mental stimulation may then add more load to the coping process because it also raises arousal level and may then help to lead on to depression. Success leads to a sense of satisfaction but failure causes frustration and may precipitate violence in association with depression.

To help the person who has risked suicide, you must know the nature of the challenges which have had to be coped with. These may be divided into two groups: (a) those which are externally determined, and (b) those which are personally, i.e., internally determined.

Externally determined strains on coping

These will represent factors which occur in the environment in which the person lives or works. Indeed, it is frequently the summation of events at work and home which brings about the exhaustion of coping. Some people seem to be born with very little coping power. They are often referred to as having inadequate personalities. Quite simple difficulties may seem to them to be gigantic. They are constantly at the end of their tether because their coping power is so low. To keep them from recurrent attempts at suicide it is necessary to surround them with metaphorical cushions to lessen the blow when they fall down. Some of them are quite intelligent and it seems so incongruous that they stumble over the smallest problems in life. They are very demanding of attention and expect someone to drop all else they are doing to rush to their aid.

Only a secure and quiet life will sustain them and this is by no means easy to arrange.

One of the most demanding of challenges in family life is a broken home. This may be a home broken by parents splitting up and thus leaving children with a continuous strain, especially if they were equally attached to both parents and so pine for the one that they are not living with. Or it may be a break-up between husband and wife or between a man and woman who have lived for some time together but not got married. The one who makes the break frequently has someone else to turn to, whereas the one left behind is likely to feel very insecure. This is especially true if he or she has few friends and no relatives near at hand.

This represents the time when befriending is most needed. They will need someone to help build some security back into their lives. Frequent contact is necessary and sometimes a strong right arm to reinforce the security. It takes some months usually to help to establish someone in a secure life once they have been left. A whole social structure of life is necessary so that the person has the stimulation of meeting friends who can share the burden of comforting and uplifting and giving support. In the case of a mother left with young children, this is particularly important. She may have no baby-sitter to let her go out in the evenings or she may never have made contact with other mothers at the child's school. The withdrawn, shy person is extremely hard to help in this way and yet she most needs the stimulation and support of a number of friends and contacts.

Family strife

This is in some ways a greater strain than the final separation. The friction in the family, however, may lead to some mental stimulation and may keep the brain sufficiently aroused to mask the underlying depression. The 'attacker' in the argument may feel stimulated by it but the person 'attacked' may be constantly frustrated and end up feeling depressed. The children in such families are often torn between the two parents.

Visiting the homes where such strife goes on may make it settle down. Often they will not argue and fight when an outsider is there. While the person who succumbs is in hospital there is a breathing space and the family given support afterwards may be able to refrain from the arguments and battles and allow peace to return. Not infrequently, the 'attacker', without the stimulation of the arguments, may begin to feel depressed some two or three weeks later when the high arousal level has come down and exposed the previously masked depression.

Helping the children from such strife-torn homes is not always so easy. First of all it is necessary to find out whether the difficulties at home have led to interference with school work. The teacher who is unaware of the home environment may interpret poorer work as just due to laziness and punish the child accordingly. It is essential to try to lower the excitement level all round if the child is to be able to cope with all aspects of life while growing up. Sometimes it is best if the child spends some weeks with a relative or friend. Even then the child may be too depressed to work at school without treatment with antidepressants.

Another aspect of family strife becomes manifest when the father has to work away from home for periods of time. Teenage children may then take advantage of his absence and become unruly. The friction generated and sometimes the retribution when father comes home may lead to breakdown of the child's coping ability. Befriending may play a very important role here in encouraging the child to obey sensible rules and allow peace to be re-established. Once again it may be several months before the child can cope without support. The long time-scale of the recovery from exhaustion of coping is frequently not appreciated and help may be withdrawn too early.

Working mothers

These are nowadays common even when they have young children. With modern devices to facilitate housework, mothers would feel bored and unfulfilled without something to do. However, the mother who comes home after her children arrive from school may not be aware of what is happening in the child's life. When children come home from school there is a short time when they are bubbling over with excitement to recite all the good and bad things which have gone on that day. By an hour later, they will be playing or doing homework and not bother to tell their parents. Thus a child's life may become disturbed without the parents understanding the reasons.

Another aspect of mothers working full time, or the 'twilight shift' from 6 pm to 10 pm after spending all day with toddlers, is that they get tired more easily and have less patience with husbands and children. Friction may be set up at these times and go on to more violent arguments. A mother who takes part in the social life of the works may find this stimulating and enjoyable but she may get worn out by it and end up desperate. After attempting suicide, it is important that she spend some weeks at least under less of a strain. She needs constant attention over this time, not only to recover from the desperation which exhausted her coping power but also to help her through the difficult time when she does not know who knows and who does not that she has risked her own death. Wondering what people will think and say is a very difficult problem when she first comes home.

In a few cases the strains within the family become intolerable. It may be precipitated by a worn out working mother, it may be started by a severely anorexic daughter who not only resists and resents the struggles of the family to make her eat, but also is likely in her disgruntled state to pick arguments and fights with any one of them. The father may then take solace in the local public house and may return in a vicious mood. The children learn to get out of his way and go to bed before he arrives but the mother may be the butt of his verbal abuse or his fist. There is a limit to the battering that a wife can take and not a few attempt suicide in desperation. They need particular care when they leave hospital and sometimes they need help in obtaining appropriate legal restrictions on their husbands. Not infrequently the husband may need help but this is usually medical rather than befriending.

The husband may take the overdose because of the severity of the challenges to his coping ability. In these cases he is rarely a drunkard but is more likely to be an over-working man, exhausting himself for his family and losing a great deal of sleep under the mental strain. As his coping nears its limit, he may strike out regardlessly and later be filled with remorse when he realises what he has done. He may well need a great deal of help subsequently and perhaps require advice in getting his affairs into a state that will not exhaust him.

Personally determined strains on coping

At first thought it may seem strange that anyone should contrive to get themselves to a point where they could no longer cope with challenges of their own making. Clearly this depends upon the person's personality. The people who do this tend to be those with a determined, driving personality. Often they are perfectionists and drive themselves on and on to achieve the high goals they set themselves. They tend to be ambitious, want to do well in examinations and climb the socio-economic ladder to the top. Whether they achieve all these things or not depends upon their innate ability but frequently they push themselves way beyond what they have any hope of achieving.

Some of these people have been labelled type A behaviour people and they are known to have a higher incidence of coronary thrombosis (heart attack) than the more placid, less driving type B people. The strain of driving themselves to the limit of tolerance may lead to the frustration of failure. At that time they may feel their coping power is exhausted and take an overdose of drugs, trying to escape from their own failure. They are quite difficult to handle afterwards. The overbearing ambition is so difficult to curb. At every turn they are trying to escape from the helpful support of friends and relatives. The frustration of their unsatisfied desires makes them reject the very help they most need.

Self-starvation

Some of the high-driving people are made to develop this characteristic rather than being born with it. This is sometimes true of one group of perfectionists, the women who starve themselves and have anorexia nervosa. This is much commoner than it used to be and is mostly in teenagers and those in their early twenties. In severe cases their lives become stereotyped and they may become obsessed with tidiness. Everything has to be very precisely in place, books with their edges parallel to the edge of the table or shelf on which they lie. Nothing can be left lying about, it must be picked up and put precisely in place. Their handwriting is meticulously neat, on a straight line with every letter identical all over the page.

Their starving usually starts because they are a bit overweight or because of the fashion for girls to be slim. They soon discover that when made to eat by the family they feel less well and are less able to work. In fact starvation excites the brain and raises arousal level. It is this that they come to be dependent on. A mother will sometimes describe how her daughter changed over a year from being a happy, carefree, untidy girl to being a solemn, overworking, excessively tidy but irritable and self-willed person whom she hardly recognised. Some anorexics push themselves to the limit of tolerance and the high arousal of starvation may then fail to mask the underlying depression. Frustration with their failure to achieve what they, and perhaps others, expect of them may lead to self-injury. They are not easy to treat but it has to be by people outside the family because so often the strain on all members of the family brings it to breaking point. Their iron willpower gets them past the normal point of hunger until appetite is totally suppressed. The same iron will defies all but the stoutest heart in getting them over this illness successfully. The severest ones have to be in hospital anyway but many can be treated outside hospital if the family gets enough support. Since 75% start crash dieting in the year they are working for an important examination, it is often very difficult to help them until their examinations are over.

In recent years self-imposed starvation has become much commoner among married women. These are women usually in their thirties who previously have not been anorexic. Many are on the verge of depression and then discover that not eating causes mental excitement and they then refuse to go back to eating. Since they are sometimes so near to depression it is not surprising that they get desperate at times, especially since friction is set up between them and their husbands because starvation causes total loss of libido.

Sexual problems

Friction between sexual partners is one of the commonest

causes of self-injury. Overwork is an important factor in the loss of libido by women or the onset of impotence in men. Loss of libido commonly occurs in married women who take on mentally demanding jobs. She may be a secretary to a busy executive or a woman doing an open-ended job in the commercial world. They feel the mental reward of success, sometimes aided by financial rewards, and go on striving despite the needs of their family. Few husbands can understand the progressive loss of interest in lovemaking and tend to assume that they have a rival in the office. Friction mounts to arguments and perhaps to open warfare in the home till the woman, in desperation, risks killing herself. An alternative version of the same theme is the precipitation of a crisis when the woman finds that her husband is paying court to another woman.

Teenage love-affairs have been suggested as being of much greater importance nowadays compared to years ago. In fact rows between a boy and girl rarely lead to attempted suicide unless there are other factors which had been eroding the coping ability for some time before. Indeed, the friction leading to the row or the break-up is often a reflection of the fact that one or other of the couple was under such a strain as to cause the irritability and intolerance of early depression. It is essential in befriending such youngsters to find out all the other pressures in their lives which may be of more vital importance than the row which was only the trigger.

Stimulating arousal to mask depression

The effect of starvation in stimulating the arousal of the brain and thereby masking depression has already been referred to. The starving girls may not know this at the outset but they certainly use the increased arousal to facilitate greater mental agility. This was first described by those studying professional fasters at the beginning of this century.

All the techniques used to stimulate arousal level carry the potential danger that the constant high arousal will lead to the development of an underlying depression. As a result of frustration or a fall in arousal level the person may then take an overdose of drugs. Alcohol is a well-known agent which, taken in greater amounts than usual, will lower arousal and make the person aware of depression.

The stimulation used to raise arousal level varies greatly. Probably one of the commonest is the intense noise at many discotheques. It has been shown that noise of this intensity can make the brain more efficient if it is already fatigued by loss of sleep. To those not accustomed to the noise it may be painful to be present: deterioration in hearing occurs in those who are constantly exposed to such a noise. The mental excitement produced by this intensity of noise could well mask depression for a time. Eventually this, like so many other artificial mental stimuli, may lead to depression becoming obvious and then a slight trigger could initiate self-injury.

Some of the stimuli used by adolescents and young adults to mask depression are not so innocuous. Challenging authority is a device which some younger people have used. Perhaps the challenge of parental authority is one of the mildest of such stimuli and a number of young people clearly use it. This may take the form of damage to parental property, usually in such a way as not to be caught. It may be more dramatic as with breaking ornaments, doors or windows. It may be particularly used by teenagers when they have no father living with them or he is intermittently working away from home. It may be either the child or the mother who succumbs to the strain, usually when the father returns and inflicts retribution. These teenagers have invariably been under pressures of a variety of sorts and have intermittent depression. Initially they learn by accident that producing excitement (good or bad) masks depression and they then pursue a course of repeated events to raise arousal level. Almost always the depression becomes progressively more severe until it cannot easily be masked. Coping power is then near the point of exhaustion and self-injury is easily triggered.

These situations are quite difficult to handle, partly because the desire to challenge the parent to raise arousal becomes almost an addiction. More particularly they are difficult without the use of antidepressants for the teenager and often the mother as well. Strong support for the child by the befriender will be needed for many months. Discussion of the primary challenges which produced the depression in the first place is essential.

At school, challenging authority can be much more effective in terms of stirring up excitement. There may be only one or two children in a class who start a disturbance but the other children are only too glad to join in the stimulating experience. Clearly the success of this type of activity depends upon the attitude of the teacher. The strictest ones are rarely challenged because the response tends to be so fast that little excitement is caused and it is overwhelmed by the fear of severe punishment. In some classes, however, total chaos can be produced day after day so that practically no work gets done. Eventually punishment by the school and the parents helps to build the underlying depression to the point where it cannot be masked and it is then that the ring-leader may take an overdose of drugs.

Support has to be given for a long time but it is more effective if the depression is treated with antidepressants. The original underlying depression is usually related to problems at home or between boy and girl friends. Family support may be needed to resolve the problem.

Finally, the challenge may be to the law when stealing, damaging property, mugging, fighting and real violence are undoubtedly used by some young people to raise arousal level. Frequently they have had a prolonged time with multiple difficulties in life such as broken homes or intense friction at home, etc. Few of them would be expected to appeal for support by befrienders because the law and the probation service often take care of them. However, other people in the family may well be driven to depression by the child's activities and then attempt suicide. Helping such a family is a difficult and long-term job but there may well be a member of the family who needs it and could benefit by it.

Conclusions

Those who engage in self-injury are desperate at the time they do it. Primarily they wish to escape from circumstances that they feel they cannot possibly cope with. The final trigger may be relatively trivial and after an hour or two the person may see a way to cope and then ask for help. This should not lead one to think that the original act was not genuinely one of desperation. They need to escape from the challenge: they do not necessarily intend to die but they are sufficiently desperate that they will take the risk.

Constant challenges cause initial mental arousal but as coping ability fails, depression sets in. Good excitement and bad excitement are additive in this mechanism. In befriending these people, it is necessary to understand the long course of time over which things build up and the long time it takes to facilitate peace and security until coping powers return completely to normal.

Of all felicities, the most charming is that of a firm and gentle friendship. It sweetens all our cares, dispels our sorrows, and counsels us in all extremities.

SENECA

Helping people in anxiety – H. J. WALTON

A person in adulthood feels 'good' to the extent that his relations with his parents were satisfactory. A person who had bad relations with a parent will be prone, throughout life, to experience spells of 'bad' feelings: self-criticism, inferiority, depression or anxiety. In this sense the exact nature of a person's associations with his parents remain embedded in him and are a source of feeling states which can occur to him throughout adulthood.

The people we see in crisis, therefore, talk to us about their present social relationships, their own family members, and at length also about relationships they had with their parents.

A person communicates with other people by means of speech. He communicates with himself by thinking. Thought is internal behaviour. In an interview we enable the person we are helping to give us access to his internal behaviour, by asking him to tell us about his thoughts.

In our attempt to understand behaviour through talking to a person, a double task faces us. We have to understand the person in the first place, and then we have to comprehend the situation in which he finds himself. When his crisis is the result of external difficulties or pressure, we can talk of *press*, as when someone loses an important person through death. When the crisis is the result of internal pressures inside the troubled individual, we can speak of *stress*. Such internal stress can be produced by thoughts in a person's mind, by feelings such as anger or resentment, or by impulses such as sexual urges which trouble the person but which he cannot allow full expression.

A useful way of looking at people in crisis may be by assuming that when they contact us they are disturbed by painful inner tension: they suffer from anxiety which has reached an insupportable level. Anxiety is caused by the human environment. It is a mood of fear which puts out of action a whole range of normal skills and functions. An anxious person does not attend adequately to his environment, does not notice things, makes errors, is forgetful. Generally, anxiety serves to disorganise ordinary behaviour.

Anxiety can increase in intensity to produce a state of terror. If a person is appropriately predisposed, there is a wide range of life events which can precipitate a state of anxiety.

Being rejected by another person is one: as when an employee is told that his work is not good enough, or a husband tells his wife that her housekeeping does not satisfy his expectations. (Perhaps his standards are over-conscientious, ingrained in him by an excessively perfectionist mother when he was young.)

The other person may precipitate anxiety in our client or patient by more clear-cut aggression or hostility, making threats which endanger the security of the person who consults us. It can be, however, that there is no other person prominently implicated; instead it may be a person's own thoughts which precipitate anxiety in him: a mother suffering from fearfulness that she is not good enough to care for her child and will inadvertently perpetrate some harmful or even fatal accident. Thoughts connected with sex are often extremely distressing to people, and if we get from them details about their past lives, it is clear how the conflict state about sex arose. They need to express their responses of loving and physical tenderness, but there are forbidding images or memories lodged in their minds which forbid such natural expressions of love.

We arrive at mature forms of sexuality only in adulthood, passing through phases which society considers abnormal, indeed will not recognise as customary or common at certain stages of life. We forget the devious paths by which adolescents arrive at mature sexuality.

The person who contacts us will usually be in a state of excessive anxiety. This is a painful inner state, a pervasive sensation of fear which is uncomfortable and in extreme cases may be intolerable. Anxiety is so distressing a state that, when it is severe, the sufferer will seek to reduce the painful tension, sometimes in ways which lead him to suffer great harm.

There are various kinds of anxiety, with three main types. The importance of distinguishing the type of anxiety lies in the fact that for each type a different kind of approach is required.

A person may have extreme, massive anxiety because he fears he will be suddenly isolated, or because he is suddenly overwhelmed with self-reproach or self-loathing, or because he dreads that some harm is about to befall him in relation to his body.

The first type of anxiety, the dread of isolation, occurs when a person is suddenly deprived of the support of another person upon whom he had been more deeply dependent than perhaps he knew. He may lose the protecting person through death; a woman may lose the husband on whom she is emotionally dependent because he leaves her for another woman; a person may never have married in order to retain the protectiveness of a parent, and be precipitated into an anxiety attack if the parent withdraws affection or support.

This type of separation anxiety has been studied in small children who are taken from parents when admitted to hospital; but you can also see very similar reactions in adults, say in a woman whose husband leaves on a business trip overseas, or in someone whose more emotionally robust marriage partner becomes ill.

The second type of anxiety, the anxiety of self-disgust, is different. Healthy people have a reasonable appreciation of their own attainments; they tell themselves that, considering the obstacles they have encountered, they have acquitted themselves fairly adequately. But the anxiety which comes from an unhealthy conscience leads a person to think that he has failed, that he betrayed all the trust reposed in him, that he is a disgrace to those who had believed in him. This type of anxiety leads the person to say to whoever is approached for help: 'Please don't let my mother or father hear of this.' Such a person will figuratively beat his head, overcome with self-hatred and abnegation. They may say that they deserve only condemnation or punishment. Some may actually punish themselves, taking their chastisement in their own hands. These people are flayed by their consciences. Psychologically they have, as part of their minds, attitudes of self-disgust. These attitudes are seen by psychiatrists as stemming from hatred or criticism or rejection experienced during growing up. Disliked by a parent, they have come to carry for ever, as part of their mentality, the inner reflection of what was once directed upon them from the censorious parent. Now it has become a part of the self. Any criticism they evoke, a failure of their efforts, or even a reproof uttered by someone in the heat of anger, suddenly lights up their own stores of self-criticism.

Only someone who has experienced the horror of being alone in a state of terror while the full light of consciousness plays relentlessly over all the weakness, failures, omissions and faults, can understand the fear which may be felt by somebody who regards himself as beyond contempt. Often such a person, when seeking help, is in an extreme dread that he has failed, that he is an outcast and would be despised if only people knew.

We recognise that when a person seeks our help for anxiety of this self-despising variety we will probably find in his life history a parent who was not able to feel appropriate affection for him. This parent is then retained in his mind throughout life as a sort of inner assailant, who can undermine him, bring him down, humiliate him. His precarious self-esteem drops to an agitatingly low level when in addition he encounters criticism or rejection in his current experience with other people.

The third type of anxiety, dread of physical damage, may be illustrated by its expression in a young man: 'Lately I go to bed many nights haunted by the fear that I won't wake up the following morning. I can assure you this fear of dying is torture to go through.'

The person is suddenly struck with terrible certainty by a fear that his heart is diseased, or that he has a cancer. People anxious in this way, overcome by a fear of some serious physical affliction, are likely to seek medical reassurance directly, so they are more prone to have their first recourse to doctors than to any other sort of helping person.

To give first aid to people with these varying types of anxiety calls for very different responses in the helping person. The individual with separation anxiety needs substitute company from a friend or a relative, or hospital care. The person with conscience anxiety, convinced of his worthlessness, needs a personal response which will revive his self-esteem. To protect and provide comfort and care for him, as advocated for the earlier type of separation anxiety, may only convince him of his worthlessness. The person with the third type of anxiety, fear of bodily dissolution, usually needs medical attention as a first step, before tracing out with him what the roots of his physical panic were.

While we may approve of the wisdom of those in trouble who seek help, they themselves may consider their help-seeking despicable. Jerome Frank has demonstrated that one of the changes occurring in people who are successfully treated by psychiatrists is their greater effectiveness in getting help for themselves when they feel troubled. Some people approaching us will show, as part of their personality disturbance which has not yet been improved by treatment, a great hesitancy in asking for help. Many of our clients or patients will reach us only when the extremity of their distress has pushed them over this inner barrier against asking for aid. They will often be ashamed and apologetic at this weakness, as they see it, this lapse into open admission of lack of independence. Many will not come to see us until their distress has driven them to contemplate suicide.

No receipt openeth the heart but a true friend, to whom you may impart griefs, joys, fears, hopes, suspicions, counsels and whatever lieth upon the heart to oppress it, in a kind of civil shrift or confession.

FRANCIS BACON

Coping with clients under sixteen – JOHN ELDRID

There has been a marked increase in the number of very young clients (fifteen years and under) contacting The Samaritans. Whilst it is an important principle of our work that we regard all clients as human beings irrespective of age or problem, it is useful to recognise that clients vary considerably in their approach, and our reactions vary according to what is presented.

When a fourteen-year-old rings up for the first time he or she may present what may appear to be a trivial problem about which to ring The Samaritans. He or she may complain of being afraid to go to school because of bullying or it may be that the parents do not like children staying out late. He or she may make the approach amidst giggles and laughing. It may be a general kind of enquiry about finding a club or information about knowing when you are pregnant or how to get an abortion. How do we react? We must treat the call very seriously because the giggling approach is more likely to be a cover-up for shyness. The worry about other girls or boys is likely to be only the tip of the iceberg. Samaritans must recognise that teenagers do not find it easy to be articulate about their problems, so they will have a struggle to verbalise their feelings and worries. Older people, particularly in their late twenties to fifties, do not on the whole find it so difficult to speak of their troubles, but from the fourteen-year-old we can expect initially the rather typical problems of anxiety about parents not understanding and so on, yet once you get the confidence of the girl or boy you may discover they are frequently away from school presenting false absentee notes, and that they are terrified to speak to their parents. You may be surprised to learn he or she would like to make a go of it at school and longs for someone with whom their problems can be discussed. In addition to the worry about bullies at school you may discover the parents are fighting most of the time or a break-up of the marriage is imminent – or conversely the parents may get on well, but because they are so anxious to see Johnny do well he feels depressed about letting them down, and so does not tell them the truth.

As in most cases it is the last straw that breaks the camel's back; here it could be bullying at school or breaking friends, but there is generally a big build-up behind it. We in The Samaritans should recognise that it is always a serious step to telephone us, so we have no reason to assume that the caller is not feeling desperate. It is not uncommon for young people to experience a very sudden sense of loss and depression, so that for them at the time the situation may seem quite hopeless. The feelings of young people are intense, so they are likely to be very elated at one moment with a dramatic drop to sadness and possible depression. This is one of the reasons why it is most essential for us in The Samaritans to listen to what is said and to note what is not mentioned. The assessment of these situations is by no means easy, and requires good consultation in the Branch. Some doctors and social workers are particularly concerned that much childhood and teenage depression goes unnoticed. Suicides do occur in this age group; whilst this was being written a thirteen-year-old boy killed himself in London.

Clients in this age group will be very sensitive about confidentiality, and whilst they seem mostly to have heard that The Samaritans can be trusted to keep confidences, they will be very cautious at the outset. It is therefore most important not to take any action without the client's consent. This may arouse feelings of anxiety in some about the best not being done in the end for the child; and some may feel just a little frustrated waiting upon the permission of a fourteen-year-old before taking what seems to the volunteer the obviously desirable action.

Some adults have very genuine reactions of anxiety about the need to inform parents or school – in fact the commitment to maintaining confidentiality may be more sorely tested in relation to a fourteen-year-old client than with a middle-aged man on the run for murder or some sex offence. But it is essential for us not to break confidence with the client if we are going to be a means of helping him feel it is good to be alive. The maintaining of this confidence will not only affect him positively, but will encourage others of the same age group to contact us. Once we have built up a good relationship, the boy or girl is usually more than happy for us to contact school or parents or whatever, and if they do not give permission it is for a good reason. As The Samaritans are offering a safety-valve whereby pent-up emotional conflicts can be safely released, it is more than likely that the boy or girl will be capable of taking the next positive steps without the need for Samaritan intervention at home or at school.

If we do have occasion to speak with parents or school teachers we must be careful not to blame them for the situation. They may feel guilty about their little Johnny being so desperate that he had to go to the Suicide people, so they may at first react aggressively. We must listen also to them. With teachers it is generally easier, but it is important to recognise that we are seeking their co-operation and guidance and not telling them how to run their school. Many teachers are pleased with our interest and will often end up by unloading on to us their worries about the particular case and many similar ones.

This increase in our calls for children and teenagers does not indicate that everything is worse than it was in our day – it is simply that young people today know that there are a number of helping agencies available to assist people with problems. They get quite a lot of information about the work of The Samaritans in school and often write up accounts of our work as a special project, so it is not surprising they turn to us. Also present-day society does to some extent encourage people to express their anxieties whatever their age group, and so many more people, instead of suffering in silence as they may have done in the past, now ring The Samaritans. That's what we are for.

Parents are the last people who should have children.

A Teacher

Problems of the middle-aged – CHAD VARAH

When my triplet sons were small, Michael would often point out to visitors that he was the eldest and David, with equal pride, that he was the youngest, if only by five hours, which left Andrew with little claim on any admiring exclamations that might be offered. But one day he announced, 'Well *I*'m the middlest.'

The special difficulties of the elderly receive almost as much discussion as those of 'youth' and much more than the exciting period Miss Jean Brodie called her 'prime' or that period, practically a synonym for dullness and mediocrity, called middle age. 'I'm getting middle-aged, I suppose' usually means 'it'll be downhill the rest of the way to the grave'. Yet it is from people in this age group that most of the beneficial contributions to our society come. Between forty and retiring age, both men and women tend to know who they are and what they have to give, and to be more conscientious and less likely to be distracted from their duties than when they were young. If they have any skill to offer, it is likely to be at its most practised, and though experience may teach people to keep on making the same mistakes, it is more likely to be a safeguard against bright ideas that won't work.

The middle-aged frequently hold those positions which are with good reason called 'senior', and are in most cases married, with children who are already young adults. If they are owner-occupiers of their houses, this adds to their authority and standing in the community. Women are mostly not yet widowed, and may well be able to choose between paid and voluntary work and at some stage decide how much of their lives to give to the enjoyment of grandmotherhood.

Why, then, safely beyond most of the uncertainties and confusions of youth, and not yet suffering a tremendous weakening of their powers, do so many men and women illustrate the distinction between prime and middle age?

Whilst the middle-aged may suffer any type of problem, just like other age-groups, the commonest ones that bring people to The Samaritans concern occupation and relationships, including sexual relationships.

It is well known that in our society the over-forties, particularly men, find it difficult to change jobs or to get a new one if redundant or dismissed. In those occupations which provide a pension, it is not economic to take on someone who after only a few years of service will become entitled to a pension. Furthermore, a certain seniority in age goes uncomfortably for all concerned with a junior position: those who would be quite willing to take instructions from a younger colleague may find the latter objecting. Junior positions are also likely to have lower rates of remuneration, insufficient for the commitments of many middle-aged persons.

The chief obstacle to one of the over-forties getting a new job may be his/her disinclination to lose status by accepting a position which attracts less social respect than the previous one, even if as well, or better, paid. To reconcile a person imprecisely but impressively described as an 'executive' to becoming (say) a postman may well be a counselling rather than a befriending job, though since it does not require any forbidden 'probing' questions, an experienced befriender may casually introduce into a conversation innocent enquiries about what would relations, neighbours, former colleagues think about the change, and what effect might it be expected to have on the person's health to be humping a bag of mail door-to-door instead of being deskbound when not sitting in a car on the way to sit in front of a television set. Not so long ago, Americans were proud of the number and variety of the occupations they had had experience of before becoming sufficiently prominent for anyone to listen to the catalogue, but increasing specialisation and the need for relevant qualifications and/or union recognition seem to have inhibited this vocational mobility.

Anyone who feels himself/herself to be on the scrap heap

clearly needs a sympathetic listener, but may feel that the restoration of some self-respect leaves the problem unsolved. It is true that Samaritans do not pretend to solve problems, but in those cases where nothing less is acceptable they are well advised not to begin befriending without making this clear. Happily, there are cases where the morale-boosting by the volunteer enables the client to see his/her strengths and weaknesses more realistically and therefore to attempt some initiatives on the basis of actual resources, but such a satisfactory outcome cannot be guaranteed. It is good if the client decides not to demand what no one is likely to offer, but not good if he/she is determined not to settle for what is possibly available.

Change of lifestyle can be tricky to adjust to, and if it is not self-chosen it can lead to depression. One of the things to look out for is depression hidden behind an array of seemingly intractable problems.

It is wise for a person to take up new interests as he/she becomes incapacitated for the enjoyment of former ones, but enthusiasts should beware of trying to 'sell' their own interests to clients, and patiently draw out what the person might really wish to explore. There are so many exciting things to do or study, but it has to be remembered what a subjective word 'exciting' is.

Relationships in middle age often cause difficulty: the children no longer listen respectfully, if at all, and a spouse may have so completely triumphed in the long battle to have his/her own way as to leave the other beaten and resentful. Some spouses have become more and more strangers to one another as the things for which familiarity has bred contempt are progressively concealed, and others may have become so used to one another that instead of being as comfortable together as folded arms or crossed knees, they have become so boring that all sexual attraction is lost.

Much has been written about the menopause in women, and in the last decade also about the equivalent some ten years later in the male, but writing about it doesn't make it go away nor are all results of studies about the condition taken in by the general public so as to make them more understanding. The woman suffering tiresome symptoms of the change of life should seek the medical help which is now available, and then settle down to enjoy sex without fear of pregnancy, if she has or can find a partner.

One of the kindest things one can do in discussing their difficulties in life with women in their forties is to make no mention of the word 'menopause', for such women are sick of everything being put down to this, and of being expected to be difficult or unwell. Let any diagnosis come from them or their doctor.

The so-called male menopause isn't the termination of reproductive ability, which may continue in a centenarian, but an almost obsessive attempt to recover lost youth by doing things the young do, particularly in their supposed sexual freedom and prowess. The realisation that one of a man's two feet is in the grave makes him painfully aware of what he missed when the half-way mark was still well in the future. He will sometimes go to extraordinary lengths to feed the illusion that he is as virile as ever he was, and because he is more patient, more determined and more practised, he may in fact be able to enthrall some young thing for a while, to the distress of his self-righteous wife and the embarrassment of his children, possibly older than his mistress. We have to recognise that if he is the client, he is the one with whom we sympathise, not other people who may be inconvenienced by his antics. Ageing and death are not amusing, nor must we find ludicrous the expedients of human beings to take their minds off these horrors, escapable only by dying young, suddenly.

Befriending is often of great help in cases of this kind. The mere fact that the Samaritan does not utter irrelevancies implying disapproval such as 'and you have those three lovely grand-daughters' is a relief – one client who was told this by his meenister replied curtly, and most aptly, 'I don't fuck them.' Acceptance of the difficulty as a real one, common to most middle-aged humans, is therapeutic. It's been known for a man to persist in behaviour all his family and friends denounce as ludicrous and unreasonable, and on being befriended by a Samaritan who accepts his behaviour as totally understandable and quite intelligently directed towards getting what he in fact wants, has decided to desist from it on the ground that the price other people are paying for what of course he wants is unacceptably high.

In middle age a man who has lived a heterosexual life with no penchant for homosexuality or the deviations may find that with waning powers or decreasing opportunities, neglected yearnings from his youth catch up with him. If these combine with loneliness and depression, he may engage in some form of sexual behaviour which causes scandal or even gets him in trouble with the police. Or he may simply despise himself for lusts which his conditioning does not allow him to satisfy. In either case he may become suicidal, and it is important for Samaritans to recognise this, to take his romantic longings seriously, and to recognise that those who are 'living, and partly living' may choose death because what they are afraid of is death.

Now, at this moment in time, or at any moment, we're only a cross-section of ourselves. What we really are is the whole stretch of ourselves, all our time, and when we come to the end of this life, all these selves, all our time, will be us – the real you, and the real me.

J. B. PRIESTLEY, *Time and the Conways*

Care of the elderly – PETER JEFFERYS

Many elderly people have never heard of The Samaritans; if they have, they may not think they would be able to help or may not be comfortable with a telephone; our first contact may, therefore, be with the carer, often with needs of his or her own, rather than direct with the client. This in turn may add the dimension of conflicting loyalties.

It is also important to remember that the process of ageing varies with individuals, whose needs are not static, who do not necessarily conform to a pattern and who are not necessarily ill, although they are likely to be more vulnerable to physical and mental illness. But we tend to forget that the majority of elderly people are well and happy.

Assuming, however, for our purposes that there are difficulties, the first is likely to be in communication itself. Loss of hearing calls for good, slow diction; confusion for simplicity. As with all clients, we must be careful to relate to their own experience, ask relevant questions and acknowledge, rather than deny, their feelings even if little or nothing can be done to ease them at the time.

Unfortunately not all clients are capable of accepting the reassurance they seek, for even if given it may be pushed out of the way by irrational beliefs or chronic anxiety about, for example, the electricity bill or who will do the washing. Or there may be paranoid delusions about, for example, harmful rays being poured through the walls. Apart from avoiding argument, there is little to be done apart from maintaining contact and admitting honestly that we are not being much help at present.

Confusion may mean different things to different people, so we should be careful to establish exactly what we are talking about. Where confusion in the medical sense exists, it may have different causes. Stress may lead to the client feeling harassed; severe depression to bewilderment and getting out of touch with reality; bereavement may be a factor; physical illness may have caused actual changes in the brain; chronic, usually progressive loss of memory and skills may spell the irreversible advent of dementia.

An elderly client may make statements which are, on the face of it, unlikely to be true – for example 'I must go now, my mother will be expecting me.' No purpose will be served either by entering into arguments or by appearing to accept such signs of confusion without question. Some might consider the art of distraction to be slightly dishonest but its practice may stop the client leaving immediately and supply an opportunity for relief.

Loneliness is common among those aged 75 and over, although of course it can be suffered at any age. In one survey among people over 75, half to two-thirds complained of having suffered from it within the last month, a quarter of them severely. The older one gets, the more likely one is to live alone, and over 50% of women over 80 live alone. Such loneliness is more intense where there is significant recent loss, and the highest level of distress about loneliness was felt by – and this may at first seem surprising – those in residential care. It is perhaps less surprising when we remember that it is often the most difficult personalities who go into residential care, and that residents may well be sharing rooms and other facilities with those whom they would hardly have chosen as friends and therefore come to be 'lonely in a crowd'. In addition, those in residential establishments may well have suffered more losses which in turn precipitate feelings of loneliness.

Elderly people are more liable to suffer loss than any other age group, although they often manifest the most remarkable resilience and toughness. Loss may be of various sorts, for example, financial; of a home, resulting in sharing or going into residential care; of status, after retirement; of physical and mental health, perhaps with confusion and loss of memory; of friends and partners; of independence and mobility. After suffering loss, people are more prone to depression, and especially if they have suffered from it earlier in life or where there appears to be a genetic predisposition.

Despite – or perhaps because of – the fact that one of the major losses in old age is of friends and partners, very few over the age of 75 are frightened of dying and it is much less a taboo subject than with younger people. Of course bereavement remains a major trauma, as with all age groups, but most older people cope with it remarkably well and adopt a very matter of fact approach to death.

Individual personality will exert a significant influence on the circumstances of the individual elderly person. Personality itself is usually stable and changes little (although traits may become more pronounced in older age), and it is as rich and variable among older as among younger people.

Another aspect of old age which is of great concern to doctors is, of course, neurotic illness. The incidence of anxiety neurosis is highest in the elderly, many of whom are housebound because of it, and worries about bills, bowels, illness etc. may be chronic or acute. Chronic hypochondria is both common and hard to live with and may well cause carers to suffer from stress.

Depression is also common among the elderly. Its onset may be sudden or gradual and it may be mild or severe. In a survey carried out among elderly people who had recently been admitted to a general hospital, one third had experienced depression within the previous year. For many, of course, the reason for going into hospital – often loss of some sort – was associated with the depression. One in ten of those over 65 in the community suffer from depression, and one in three in residential homes. Some illnesses such as Parkinsonism, arthritis if there is pain and loss of mobility, chronic heart and chest diseases and strokes limiting mobility may all lead to depression. (Brain damage leading to emotional lability is in a different category.)

When assessing depression, it is as well to remember that the word is comparatively recently in vogue: elderly people who do not understand it may deny it, and it may be better to ask if they are miserable, or find life not worth living, than to ask if they are depressed.

Among the elderly, agitated depression is the most

common form, often associated with anxiety which is worse in the morning, sleeplessness, appetite and weight loss. There may be delusions of illness or guilt, or a pathetic depression, which can sometimes be confused with dementia.

The outlook for the depressed elderly patient is not good. Those under 70 fare better, and depression of sudden onset is more likely to respond to treatment. Those with a history of illness do less well. Only about one third of those admitted to hospital do well in the long term (bearing in mind that four-fifths of them will have undergone some recent major change). One third may not be helped by hospitalisation and the remainder may become ill again within two or three years.

Suicide is a major risk among the elderly, particularly for men, those with a drink problem, or those living alone. Admission of the intent and plans of how to carry it out are more likely in this group. The most common method is by an overdose of drugs. Those who have tried and failed are more likely to succeed next time. Hospitalisation may help, as may social support, removal of drugs, establishing a good professional relationship, active treatment and social support.

Another major risk is self-neglect, not only in terms of eating but also financially. Again, those living alone are most vulnerable and hardest to reach.

Relapse into depression is an ever-present risk: the chronically depressed may become overdependent and the manipulative may alienate their carers, isolate themselves and therefore increase their risk of successful suicide.

Abuse by carers is, of course, well known. The worst risk has been found to be in a three-generation family, where there is usually a woman in the middle who is being pulled three ways.

Samaritans should be alert both to the problems of the elderly and of those who care for them, as well as to the difficulties of reaching them. It may be that with this group you have a right to intrude. Many local services can be improved and there are benefits to be gained by sharing experiences with other groups. But be sure that the same criteria are applied as with younger clients: they should always be treated with dignity and respect; their independence should be valued; overdependence should be avoided; they must maintain their right of choice. Beware above all talking about elderly people without including them in the conversation in a 'Does He Take Sugar?' situation.

Remember now thy Creator in the days of thy youth, while the evil days come not, nor the years draw nigh, when thou shalt say, I have no pleasure in them; while the sun, or the light, or the moon, or the stars, be not darkened, and the clouds return after the rain: in the day when the keepers of the house shall tremble, and the strong men shall bow themselves, and the grinders cease because they are few, and those that look out of the windows be darkened, and the doors shall be shut in the streets, when the sound of grinding is low, and he shall rise up at the voice of the bird, and all the daughters of musick shall be brought low; also when they shall be afraid of that which is high, and fears shall be in the way, and the almond tree shall flourish, and the grasshopper shall be a burden, and the caper-berry shall fail: because man goeth to his long home, and the mourners go about the streets: or ever the silver cord be loosed, or the golden bowl be broken, or the pitcher be broken at the fountain, or the wheel broken at the cistern. Then shall the dust return to earth as it was: and the spirit shall return unto God who gave it. Vanity of vanities, saith the preacher, all is vanity.

(Ecclesiastes xi,9–xii,8)

Bereavement – C. MURRAY PARKES

The effects of bereavement

When we look at the effects of a bereavement, there are four main areas that we have to consider.

There is *grief* itself – that is to say the psychological reaction to the loss.

There are the effects of *deprivation*. For instance, a woman who loses her husband not only suffers from the loss of her husband, but she also has to learn to live without him. She is, from then onwards, a person without a husband. She suffers not only loss but psychological starvation.

Then there is the *role change* that accompanies most losses – the fact that being a married woman, for instance, is not the same thing at all as being a widow. A person in one situation in life has to learn a new set of roles.

Attached to this is the way in which this change in role is perceived by society, particularly in the case of many losses the *stigma* which is associated with the loss. Here again, one can think in terms of loss of a person, or one can think in terms of other types of loss. For instance, an amputee – someone who loses a limb – is undoubtedly stigmatised – he becomes the recipient of sympathy. Sympathy is a very belittling thing. It is very damaging to self-respect. It's a stigma.

This involves more than a negative hostile element which undoubtedly does creep in; it includes the way in which people are frightened and embarrassed by those who are closely associated with loss, particularly where a death is involved. Every widow discovers that there are certain people who find it very difficult to talk to her, who feel somehow threatened by her, and they react in an embarrassed way.

This stigma is less obvious in our society than in many

others where the widow may come under quite severe taboos for a period after her bereavement. In one island in the Philippines the widow is not allowed to see or speak to anybody. She walks through the forest with a stick which she taps on trees to warn people that she is coming, and it is believed that even the trees she touches will die, so closely is the widow associated with the death of the person whom she survives. The same fears exist in our civilisation and I think they account for some of the tendency to ignore, avoid and blind ourselves to the needs of bereaved people.

The process of grieving

There are several factors which determine whether a person goes through the process of grieving in a healthy manner or develops one of these abnormal reactions. There are three main considerations: there is the nature of *the relationship with the dead person* and other factors influencing the magnitude of the grief itself. Here I put two things first: dependence and ambivalence. Where the relationship has been a very dependent one with the widow or widower highly involved – to the point that her whole life centred on the other person – she is particularly liable to develop a severe reaction after the loss. There is also the opposite type of relationship. The husband and wife have quarrelled a great deal and perhaps there have been times when one has actually wished the other one dead. When death wishes are gratified the survivor has a tremendous load of guilt to make up. And it sometimes happens that the survivor will do a complete about-turn and say 'I was always quarrelling with my husband, but now I realise he was right'. In order to try to put this right she will spend the rest of her life in mourning for him. There are, of course, other forms which this ambivalent attitude can take.

The second main determinant is the effect of *defence* – the defences of the bereaved person against pain and distress. Now, we all know people who are very good at defending – very good at not facing up to unpleasant fact. We know families, too, where a 'stiff upper lip' is something which is a pride. 'People don't cry in our family.' So this isn't only a personal thing. It's a cultural factor. In fact there are many cultures which place very high value on the ability to control emotions and not to break down or to cry in situations which one would expect would give rise to this. Among the widows about whom I was talking earlier, those who showed the least emotion during the first fortnight of bereavement were uniformly more disturbed three months later than the rest. It appears that one can postpone grief, but one cannot deny the need to grieve. Sooner or later it will break through, and that's why defending oneself in this way doesn't seem to be a satisfactory answer to the problem of grief.

Finally, there are the effects on the rehabilitation of the widow of *the environment* in which she finds herself, and here I would put social isolation as the commonest cause of trouble. If a person has a close warm family who stand by her at the time of bereavement, then she will find during the course of the next few years that there is something left in life, that there are people who can share her grief, and people who can bring her out of it. Socially isolated people tend to get 'stuck' with the chronic type of grief. Rather less common, but also a problem that can arise, is the bereaved person who is over-protected. The tendency for the family to take over is perhaps not a bad thing at first, but in time can tend to be unhealthy, if it goes on after the period when the widow would normally have found herself a job, gone out, and so on. This is particularly the case where there are young unmarried daughters at home who are willing to take over a large part of the role of the widow. We all know the situation that can arise here.

Grief work – Chad Varah

The most important thing Samaritans can do to help someone who has suffered a severe bereavement is to encourage them to do what has come to be called 'grief work'. This involves taking out and looking at the memories of the one who has died, whether these were good or bad, and 'working' through them a sufficient number of times for them to be accepted, assimilated, and gently put away. Nothing prevents a bereaved person from readjusting to life more than the selfish habit of most of their relatives and friends of frustrating this need by changing the subject. They pretend this is for the mourner's good, but it is to protect themselves from embarrassment or boredom. We Samaritans are willing to assist patiently with 'grief work'.

Deeply religious people are often troubled with guilt because they find themselves railing at God for having 'taken' their loved one, and then fearing divine displeasure for the 'blasphemy' of hating Him and not trusting Him to know best. They need to be assured that God understands how natural it is to yell or lash out when hurt, and that it would *really* be on the way to blasphemy to suppose that He cannot understand or forgive as well as a Samaritan.

In extreme cases a priest may help by giving the bereaved person express permission to blame God with impunity.

The last act is always tragedy, whatever fine comedy there may have been in the rest of life – we must all die alone.

BLAISE PASCAL

Befriending the homosexual – CHAD VARAH

We are all to some extent homosexual, in that we retain from that period in our childhood when we were almost entirely homoerotic a capability both for deep affection for and sexual attraction to those of our own sex even if soon after puberty we joined the vast majority who find the opposite sex more sexually exciting and desirable.

This may be illustrated by the behaviour of men or women confined in a situation when for a longish period they are cut off from the society of the opposite sex. Homosexual practice in one-sex boarding schools or in prisons or on ships at sea are no proof, by themselves, of predominant homosexual leanings on the part of the participants. Many a public school boy has had no difficulty in distinguishing between those of his sexually very active contemporaries who are 'really' homosexual, and who will be observed to continue into adult life; and those who are 'making do', and even on a short exeat will manage to get at some girl. But what of the ones who are apparently equally interested in pretty boys and their visiting sisters? And those who even in term time would rather masturbate while thinking about a girl than engage in sex play with another boy? And those who (whether with a low or high or medium sex drive) strive to avoid sexual arousal and gratification?

A bright schoolboy will come to the conclusion that just as you cannot divide the pupils in your class into 'clever' and 'stupid', because there is an infinite gradation from the sharpest to the thickest academically, so the same lot of boys cannot be divided into heterosexual and homosexual, as if you were bound to be purely one or the other, and as if there were no degrees of interest and lust. Strange, then, that he so often grows up to join the mob of foolish adults who are unaware of this fascinating spectrum, and who, like the old style Western with its goodies and baddies, label everyone 'straight' or 'queer'.

The reason why those of us who regard ourselves as wholly heterosexual are loth to admit that we retain any homosexual potential in our make-up is partly that we have not found ourselves in circumstances when this uncomfortable bit of self-knowledge was forced upon us, and partly that all the weight of conventional attitudes and our natural avoidance of the finger of scorn cause us to flinch away from any such awareness. Indeed, many of those who are, and know they are, markedly homosexual may try to deny this, to others if not to themselves. They want to live quietly without persecution, and who (except those more interested in politics than in love) will blame them if they decide not to 'come out', let alone man the barricades?

About 4% of the population, both male and female, finds sexual love-making with the same sex more acceptable than with the opposite sex, even though the latter activity may, for some, at a pinch, be feasible. What we do not know is how many of the remaining 96% deserve to be called heterosexual by a similar criterion, namely that they find sexual love-making with the opposite sex more acceptable than with the same sex (which of course includes oneself). When you cut out those who have not yet reached puberty and those who have become asexual through senility, those who cannot use sex in relationship but only in masturbation (which may possibly use another person's body to rub against), those who suffer from a deviation of aim or object (e.g. sadomasochists, exhibitionists, fetishists and transvestites, whose deviant desires may focus on the opposite *or* on the same sex), what percentage of the population is left? An educated guess is that something of the order of 40% deserve to be called heterosexual in the sense that (no doubt with some aid from fantasy) they can enjoy a *person* of the opposite sex. The distinction, if we feel bound to make one at all, is not between hetero and homo, but between those who can love with their sex and those who unhappily cannot.

Acceptance of these facts so completely that it has become

part of our natural and unthinking reaction to the information that a man or woman we encounter is alleged to be homosexual, is the only way the volunteer, whether more hetero or more homo, can befriend a homosexual. Only this attitude, which is scientific and true and humane (and therefore good and Samaritan) can enable us so to befriend the homosexual in crisis, without talking offensive nonsense about perversion or 'cure', that he or she will not only continue to live but probably find life richer for having encountered The Samaritans.

A moment's thought will convince us that a person who is homophile (i.e. capable of love-making with someone of the same sex) is not much more likely to seek the help of The Samaritans about homosexual problems than a 'heterophile' (to coin a word) is to seek our help about heterosexual problems. Both vague categories of human beings suffer from a variety of difficulties which may make their life appear unsupportable at the moment, and a person's sexual orientation will often be largely irrelevant to the sort of befriending he or she needs. Homophiles are a little more likely than heterophiles to want to mention their disposition and to find problems arising out of their belonging to a sometimes persecuted (though not nearly as blackmailable as pre-Wolfenden) minority, and they encounter greater difficulties in meeting a sufficient variety of other homophiles to be likely to find an acceptable partner with whom to set up home. The average homophile has the same need of a secure and mutually rewarding partnership as the average heterophile, and the frequently expressed allegation that 'homosexuals are not capable of lasting relationships' is untrue. What is, sadly, true is that without the support of society and the family which most marriages enjoy, homosexual partnerships may break up when disagreements or infidelities occur as easily as in the less family-integrated heterosexual cohabitations without marriage. Certainly there is often a need for a form of 'marriage counselling' for homosexuals, male or female, in partnerships, and good befriending by Samaritan volunteers may lead to this being found acceptable.

A most important thing for Samaritans to know and tell to others is that when a person has been identified as a male homosexual this does not mean that he is likely to be a pederast, i.e. to be one who gratifies his sexual desires with children. Just as the vast majority of heterosexuals prefer a nubile partner and do not try to seduce little girls, so the vast majority of homosexuals do not try or wish to seduce little boys. Because heterosexuals greatly outnumber homosexuals, far more little girls than little boys are 'interfered with' sexually.

Not all pederasts are violent attackers of strangers. The typical pedophile loves children and relates to them better than to adults and usually does no more than stroking of the genitals of related or known children. But it is understandable that even this arouses anxiety and indignation in their parents and other adults if the child mentions it. Without appearing rejecting or judgmental, Samaritans have to lead pedophiles to think about the long-term effects on the children concerned.

Let a male homosexual, Franklin E. Kameny, have the last word: 'The homosexual, in our pluralist society, has the moral right to be a homosexual . . . (and) to live his homosexuality fully, freely and openly, and to be so and to do so free of arrogant and insolent pressures to convert to the prevailing heterosexuality, and free of penalty, disability or disadvantage of any kind, public or private, official or unofficial, for his non-conformity.'

Since the time I lost him, I do but languish, I do but sorrow; and even those pleasures all things present me with, instead of yielding me comfort, do but redouble the grief of his loss. We were co-partners in all things.

MONTAIGNE

Alcoholism – DAVID DAVIES

Alcoholism is a topic which is riddled with myths and misconceptions. The one that should be disposed of first is the idea that nobody can say what an alcoholic is, but we all know one when we see one. That is quite untrue on both counts. We do know what an alcoholic is, and we don't recognise them when we see them.

All of us – all caring agencies, doctors, nurses, social workers, volunteers of all kinds – must work with alcoholics because of the sheer numbers. It is reckoned there are a million in the population. Whether you know it or not, some among your clients are alcoholics. You may not recognise them as such, but we do know what an alcoholic is and can now give guidance as to how to recognise one. It's not just 'look and see'.

First, what is alcoholism? It is essentially connected with the long-term use of alcohol, and in that respect it differs from just getting drunk, which could happen to anybody – even on the first time that he takes a drink. So that one element in the definition must be continuing use of alcohol over a period of time. Another element must be harm, and that harm could be in any of three spheres. It could be in the physical sphere, e.g. damage to the liver; or in the mental sphere, even to the extent of mental disorders which bring people into mental hospitals; and (what concerns you most) in the social sphere, which covers marital, occupational and economic aspects of life.

Of course, if somebody went into hospital with liver damage due to alcohol and came out a week or two later with his liver restored, which could happen, nobody would dream that he was clear of his alcoholism. His liability to continue drinking in the way that brought on the damage still persists, as does that aspect of him we call dependence. It is no different from dependence on other drugs which, like alcohol, are addictive. So I would suggest that a thumbnail definition which anybody can use is: continual or intermittent ingestion of alcohol leading to dependency or harm. And dependency may be of a physical kind, e.g. when a man has to take a drink first thing in the morning to steady his hand. Or it might mean that he has to take a drink then or at other times not to control any physical symptom, but simply to feel right – to feel able to face the day and do the work he has to do. We shouldn't play down psychological dependence and think that it's any less difficult to cope with than physical dependence, because with some drugs – amphetamine is one of these – there is no physical dependency, and yet dependency of a purely psychological kind on that type of drug can be just as desperate as (say) dependence on heroin.

The other myth that I'm sure everyone has heard, that alcoholics are born, is quite untrue. Alcoholics are made. Nobody is born an alcoholic. And the other thing you read in the text-books, that the cause is unknown, is also quite untrue. The cause is quite simple: oddly enough, it's alcohol. But one has to say a little more than that; it isn't just alcohol, but the continued use over a period of time of alcohol in quantities and in a frequency which engenders dependency. And this is true of all drugs of dependency, that nobody becomes dependent the first time they have the drug in a particular dose, but if there is repetition, then a sort of Rubicon is crossed when the body is no longer as it was previously, that is to say just the same after the dose as it was before. Now there is left something in the body about which we have learnt a great deal in the last couple of years. There is something left in the nervous system which makes the body keyed up and expectant of the next dose. But that only comes after a certain quantity and frequency. Now all drugs of dependency are harmless in certain dosages and certain frequencies, even if you become dependent. Coffee is a very good example. Most of us are dependent on coffee; we feel the need of it at certain times of the day, and if we don't get it we feel irritable. These are withdrawal symptoms. Very few of us develop damage due to coffee unless we have more than a certain quantity, which in the case of coffee is known to be five or six cups a day. Curiously enough, in the case of alcohol, it's known to be about five or six pints a day, or five or six double whiskies a day. Certainly at that level, physical harm can occur.

So it's possible to be dependent on alcohol and not be harmed by it. This may be a bit academic in a sense. But we must ask: Why then do only about 5% of us become harmed by alcohol? Rephrased, why do 5% drink so much as to harm themselves?

The reasons why they drink so much are fairly straightforward and we know a great deal about them. They are sociological reasons. There is pressure to drink for all of us as we grow up, as part of our lifestyle. Some families and some groups of people experience stronger pressures than others. In some occupations, like the drink trade, and waiting, and going abroad in the Army – and including medicine for some curious reason – where there is increased availability, there is an increased likelihood of this developing. And of course, where it's cheap and where there are fewer restrictions, such as lack of licensing controls.

So in the case of any alcoholic, it's possible by taking a careful history to decide which factors have played a part in his case. Then the cause of it is perfectly clear and the treatment is rational. If there's harm, one deals with the harm, and that's no different from dealing with harm in other ways. If it's social harm, then social workers and volunteers like Samaritans are handy to deal with that. If it's physical, then there are doctors, real doctors who look after the body; and if it's mental, there are psychiatrists to look after that aspect. That's not very difficult as a rule, particularly if the trouble is spotted before it has gone too far. But what really is difficult, having got the harm out of the way, is dealing with the dependency. Because dependency is a habit and habits are very, very powerful. If one has practised a habit for twenty, thirty or forty years it's very difficult to get out of the habit. But we know more these days about how to unlearn habits, and treatment of the dependency side of alcoholism has become rational and can be very effective in ways which it wasn't really before.

Well, how do The Samaritans come into all this? I suppose

the problem that comes up immediately is the question of suicide. It has been shown that among alcoholics the suicide rate is something like seventy times greater than in the population at large, and attempted suicide also is increased by about that factor. Moreover, the vast majority of alcoholics who either achieve suicide or make a non-fatal suicidal act, at the time they do the act have in fact got alcohol circulating in their blood. Because as I've said you can be an alcoholic with no alcohol circulating in your blood and go for days, weeks or months in that state, and therefore perfectly sober and in touch, but still have the propensity to lapse into your habitual drinking on certain cues or in certain situations. But in the harmful situations which are likely to present to *you*, the alcoholic is very likely also to have alcohol in his blood. So that if you can tide an alcoholic over that particular time, if you like to be with him for a few hours the next day when the alcohol has worked out of his blood, it could well be that though he is still an alcoholic, he is not in fact bent on suicide, and therefore the immediate goal should be fairly clear.

What are you to do then if you do identify the alcoholic? Perhaps one should ask *how* are you to identify him? None of the things you have been told is of any use to you, if I may say so. I should warn you that I am an iconoclast. I would suggest there are no lists of symptoms, or if there are it is because the man has reached such an advanced stage that you can spot him anyway and you don't need him to tell you the symptoms. The great thing is to keep in your mind the question: Is he harming himself by drink? All you have to determine is, in your own mind: Is he drinking enough to account for the harm he's got himself into? There might be other reasons for his harm as well, which might emerge in the course of the conversation and discussions you have with him, so that you have to keep an open mind about it. If his use of drink is not such as to make him vulnerable, simply on quantity and frequency, then that is probably as good a guide as any. Now it isn't easy to find out how much a man drinks, and the worst way is to ask him if he drinks or how much he drinks; but there are ways of finding out, simply by talking to him about his everyday life, how he spends the ordinary day, just listening – and I'm sure you're all very good at listening – and somewhere, while he's telling you about how he spends the day, something will crop up about on my way home from the pub, or to the pub, or in the bar or something, and that's as good a point as any to pick him up conversationally and get him to tell you more about how often he goes there and what he does there and so on. If you could keep a few figures in your mind, anybody who drinks on average something like five pints a day, or five double whiskies, that's roughly half a bottle of spirits (I never can work it out with wine because wine varies so much: it's probably about one and a half bottles of table wine a day) anybody who's been drinking that on an average for some months (and it's more likely years) is vulnerable. Certainly vulnerable to physical damage; and if he's vulnerable to physical damage then he's even more vulnerable to social damage, because the cost of it is enough to bring economic difficulties to many families where economically they live on the margin. Of course, if he's had treatment, and acknowledges this or volunteers it, that's a help.

A very good clue is: the surest way to find an alcoholic is to enquire about the family of a known alcoholic. It does run in families, but not in the sense in which one could indict genetic factors. It runs in families for the simple reason that families share a life style, and if the life style is what the Americans would call positive to drinking, then all the members of the family are likely to drink to a greater extent than a family where, again in the same jargon, attitudes to drinking are negative. So these are the things to look for. Of course, if a man's lost his driving licence on a drink-driving charge that's something to make you prick your ears up and think about it. Certainly if he's done it twice or if he's had high blood alcohol when doing it, that's almost diagnostic.

But what about the future? The present services are very sketchy. The Health Service has an Alcohol Treatment Unit. There's one in every health region; it's usually located in the old psychiatric hospital, which is usually well away from the urban area where the problems really occur. Of course, a man can be referred there: he can be referred to his doctor, who might refer him there. GPs vary a great deal, they tend to judge an alcoholic on whether he drinks more or less than they do, and some of the stories I hear about unhelpful general practitioners, I'm sure, are true although I'd like to disbelieve them.

There is a network of information centres growing up which actually offers advice as well as information and there are volunteers being trained, and we've been picking the brains of your own organisation and of the marriage guidance people to see how we could best train volunteers to do it. Each year now there will be increasing numbers of volunteers manning information centres, organised by the National Council on Alcoholism. There are of course religious organisations such as the Salvation Army and the AA. They tend in a particular place to cull the kind of man who is best suited for them. But there's no one way to Rome and these agencies, even though they all have a different approach, all have their uses. If a man doesn't do well with one he will quite likely do well with another.

I am arrived at last in the presence of a man so real and equal, that I may drop even those under-most garments of dissemination, courtesy and second thought which men never put off, and may deal with him with the simplicity and wholeness with which one chemical atom meets another.

RALPH WALDO EMERSON

Drug dependence – CHAD VARAH

Compulsive or addictive behaviour is likely to lead to problems for the victim, who will therefore need help. Some of the persons affected will seek this help, at some stage, from The Samaritans.

We are not concerned here with alcoholism, the most common form of gradual, non-admitted suicide in Western countries, nor with compulsive gambling or over-eating or other addiction, but with dependence on drugs.

The term 'drugs' covers a wide range of chemical preparations, solid, liquid or vaporised, which may be ingested, injected, inhaled, sniffed, rubbed on the skin, used as an enema or suppository, or surgically implanted. The vast majority of them are prescribed or self-prescribed for therapeutic purposes, though some are frequently and some occasionally misused – only the hallucinogens have no medically approved use and are therefore procured only illegally for abuse.

In common parlance, 'drugs' is a pejorative word, implying dangerous substances abused by weak-willed and disreputable persons called 'drug addicts'. Even in the sense of a substance of addiction, the victims of the commonest and arguably the most dangerous of these, nicotine, would indignantly reject aspersions on their respectability. Although this article is concerned with drugs of dependence, usually as a result of misuse, it should be mentioned that Samaritans try to preserve the neutral sense of the word, for they often have to reassure callers that they will not become 'drug addicts' by taking medicaments prescribed by a qualified doctor, even over a long period, any more than a diabetic person can be described as an insulin addict. Apart from patients with otherwise uncontrollable pain, such as those with certain forms of terminal illness, doctors rarely prescribe drugs in doses which make the patient dependent on them. Most drugs are not commonly abused and do not lead to dependence.

Among the drugs callers may have had prescribed by their GP, in alphabetical order, are those for alcoholism, for allergies, analgesics, for angina, antacids, antibiotics, anticoagulants, anti-convulsants, antidepressants, antihistamines, antihypertensics, antispasmodics, bronchodilators, corticosteroids, for diabetes, diuretics, for epilepsy, expectorants, hypnotics, inhalants, laxatives, for nausea, opiates, for rheumatism, sedatives, stimulants, tranquillisers, for ulcers, vitamins and for vomiting. Under each heading there may be several or hundreds of preparations, each with a pharmaceutical name and a proprietary one, and it would be beyond the scope of this article (or the competence of this writer) to describe their effects or the effects of an overdose of them. Samaritans who encounter overdoses of unfamiliar substances should not be tempted to act on 'a little knowledge'. The same applies to the effects of failing to take a prescribed drug in the correct dosage at the stated intervals or in the situations laid down.

Many otherwise safe drugs (in the prescribed dosage) become dangerous if combined with alcohol, or in conjunction with certain other drugs.

We are concerned here with drugs that are commonly abused. In alphabetical order, these include amphetamines, barbiturates, cannabis, cocaine, hallucinogens, inhalants, medicines containing sedatives, and opiates.

Amphetamines

Amphetamines and similar drugs powerfully stimulate the body and the mind and are therefore nicknamed 'speed'. They may still sometimes be used medically to suppress appetite for slimming. Other nicknames for such 'pep pills' are 'dexies' and 'meth', from Dexedrine (dexamphetamine tablets, yellow), and methedrine (methylamphetamine hydrochloride, white – also in ampoules). There are over a dozen common pep pills, and many less common. They are mostly taken by mouth, and make the user wakeful, alert, not hungry or tired, restless, often confused and/or irritable. After three or four hours tiredness sets in. There can be psychological dependence, with lethargy and depression after withdrawal. Regular use of amphetamines may lead to 'tolerance', i.e. in order to obtain the same effect it is necessary to take more of the drug. If there is psychological dependence, then the user most certainly will increase the dose.

With young clients in big cities showing depression and lethargy, one possible cause is the use of amphetamines.

Barbiturates

Barbiturates have the opposite effect to amphetamines. Where amphetamines tend to make the user excitable, irritable and perhaps violent, the barbiturates are hypnotics, that is to say they induce sleep, and their users are typically confused and drowsy. Like the amphetamines, barbiturates are usually used in pill form, though they may be injected, and at a time when heroin became difficult to obtain, some heroin addicts were 'fixing' with barbiturates partially dissolved – they won't dissolve completely, and some users died of the results of abscesses formed at the point of injection.

The barbiturates most commonly used and misused are Amytal, Gardenal, Luminal, Nembutal, Seconal, Sodium Amytal, Soneryl and Tuinal. They are likely to lead to both physical and psychological dependence, and it is important to remember that tolerance does not develop in the case of barbiturates to the point of preventing the abuser from being poisoned by them.

The abuser of barbiturates may well be confused with a person who is drunk – there is the same stumbling, uncoordinated movement and the same slurred speech. Barbiturates are in any case often used with alcohol, which intensifies their effect.

It is very difficult for people to give up barbiturates after they have become dependent and the withdrawal symptoms are severe. Naturally, since hypnotics depress the central nervous system and induce sleep, and reduce anxiety, cessation of their use produces insomnia and anxiety, and as phenobarbitone is used to prevent epileptic fits, serious cases of withdrawal can cause the person concerned to suffer convulsions. The physical signs of withdrawal are twitching and trembling, dizziness and nausea.

An overdose of barbiturates slows the movements and slurs the mind and dilates the pupils. If the overdose is great enough, the individual will go into a coma and die.

Because of the danger of barbiturates, doctors are being encouraged to prescribe non-barbiturate hypnotics. The ones in most common use are also the ones most abused, e.g. by being injected or by being used with alcohol: Doriden, Mogadon, Noctec and Welldorm. The most dangerous in overdose was Mandrax, before it was withdrawn. It also (like Doriden) interferes with the action of anticoagulants, if the person has to take these.

Cannabis

Cannabis includes both 'grass', also called pot or marijuana, which is the leaf and flowers of the plant, and hash, which is the resin from the plant compressed into blocks. Either can be smoked – grass by being rolled alone or with tobacco, and hash by being crumbled into tobacco. Both can be put into food or drink. If smoked, it is held in the lungs to increase the effect, which may last for several hours. 'Hash' is short for 'hashish', which strictly ought to be used not for cannabis resin but for cannabis resin mixed with opium and smoked in a pipe. This is the opiate drug of addiction which was used by the Old Man of the Mountain to keep his gang of murderers under his control – they would be made dependent on the hashish, which didn't take long, and then refused it until they had killed the designated person. This is the origin of the name 'assassin' now used for any kind of hit man, though he is more likely to be working for payment than for a supply of drugs.

'Grass' made into a cigarette, with or without tobacco, is called a 'joint', and experienced smokers draw in a good deal of air at the same time as they draw the smoke into their lungs, to increase the effect. This effect is a type of intoxication not unlike that produced by alcohol, but without hangover and with euphoria, laughter and chattiness succeeded usually not by aggression or maudlin burbling, but by quiet introspection.

There seem to be also hallucinogenic effects of cannabis, in addition to sound and colour simply being more vivid: there may be a sort of delirium, depending on the mood of the person and probably the basic character of the person at the time the use began.

It is claimed that as moderate use does not seem to produce any bad effects or physical dependence and it has not been known to cause death, possession and use of cannabis ought not to be illegal. At the time of writing, cannabis and cannabis resin are (like amphetamine) Class B drugs in the 1971 Misuse of Drugs Act. Possession of them can attract up to five years in prison and/or a fine.

The chief objection to regular use of cannabis appears to be that it seems to produce the 'don't care' attitude of the drop-out. It may well serve a useful purpose in giving young people something to rebel about and to indulge in a pretty harmless form of law-breaking. Some psychologists consider that if cannabis were legalised, something more dangerous would be taken up as an expression of rebellion against parents and Society by breaking a law.

Cocaine

Cocaine is a strong stimulant made from the coca plant of which none whatever nowadays goes into Coca-cola. It is extracted and refined into a glistening white powder and therefore is commonly known as 'snow', or by the abbreviation 'coke'. Partly because it is very expensive, and partly because it produces exhilaration and a brief pleasure in the sex organs which may even cause orgasm, it has been in recent years an 'in' drug in the United States.

It is usually taken by sniffing into the nostrils, which become damaged and stream with mucus, so that the person appears to have a continuous cold and may use very many tissues per hour. Cocaine can also be injected. Medically, it would be injected as a local anaesthetic: the present writer remembers having it at his school dentist, and round about 1928 having the dentist substitute a synthetic substance called Novocaine, which is nowadays used instead.

Apart from the destruction of the septum of the nose, continued use can produce brain damage. Dependence on it is psychological, not physical, though this has been questioned by some experts, and the usual after-effects are anxiety and some depression. There may also be hallucinations.

An even more refined and addictive form called Crack is sweeping the United States and has reached Britain.

Hallucinogens

Lysergic acid diethylamide, or LSD for short, is the most commonly encountered of the hallucinogens, but mention may also be made of dimethyltriptomene (DMT) which is related to the amphetamines but different in its effects; and mescaline.

LSD is only obtainable illegally. It has no medical use, though in the Sixties it was sometimes used as an aid in psychotherapy, and practitioners in clinical psychotherapy were instructed in the use of it.

It should be emphasised that LSD is now a Class A drug under the 1971 Misuse of Drugs Act, along with cocaine, heroin, morphine, pethedine and physeptone. This means the penalty can be up to seven years' imprisonment and/or an unlimited fine.

It should be quite clear to the reader that under the Act, you can be imprisoned or fined if it is proved that you have had a classified drug in your possession, or supplied it to another or offered to supply it to another or been concerned in supplying it to another, or have been in possession of it with intent to supply it, or have exported or imported it.

Among the classified drugs, there are many which may be legally in a person's possession because they have been medically prescribed. In these cases, it is important not to pass them to another person. But in the case of LSD, there is no possibility whatever of obtaining it legally. It is never medically prescribed. LSD is a colourless, odourless and tasteless liquid, and these facts make it all the more dangerous. It will usually be encountered in the form of microdots, though it may be in the form of the powder from which the solution is made or in the form of pills. It is almost always taken by mouth, but it can be injected or sniffed.

Hallucinogens are taken for their psychological effects: the physicai effects are not pleasurable. They include loss of appetite, nausea, insomnia, tremors, sweating and respiratory disturbance.

It is the psychological effects which are sought by the users of LSD, and which have given to the English language the word 'trip' in a specialised sense. This word suggests that the user of LSD goes elsewhere mentally for a while, and then comes back. A trip may be good or bad, but even a good one may make the person aware of material from the unconscious which may be very upsetting – this was the reason for its use in psychotherapy until this was stopped.

Enthusiasts for LSD, who have an almost religious fervour about it, speak of the aesthetic and emotional value of what they call a 'psychedelic' experience (surely 'psychodelotic' would be the correct word?). Sensory impressions are intensified and may be confused, and 'peak' experiences give to some devotees a religious sense of oneness with the universe and ineffable feelings of joy and peace. On the other hand, we should set against this the deaths which occur to users by the delusion that they can walk on water or fly out of a skyscraper window.

Persistent users may become psychotic, and those who have used LSD only once may have 'flashbacks' for years afterwards. These have particularly been encountered in victims to whom the drug has been administered without their knowledge and consent. A horrifying example was the schoolgirl to whom it was administered by the vicious boy-friend of her nasty sister in a café. The girl ran wildly along a busy street weaving back and forth amongst the traffic and narrowly escaping death, and when picked up by the police all they kept saying to her was that they wouldn't tell her parents if she said where she had procured the stuff. The only thing she wanted was to be taken *to* her parents, and she suffered terrifying experiences before being able to persuade the police to take her home. She came to the notice of The Samaritans because of brief recurrences of this bad unsought trip. Fortunately one of our consultant psychiatrists knew the appropriate treatment and was able to instruct her family doctor.

A detailed account of a more horrifying (and fatal) case may be found in the Corgi paperback *Go Ask Alice*.

Inhalants

School children in search of kicks are likely to find substances such as glues and industrial solvents which can be sniffed or inhaled and which are easily procurable and not costly. Some commercial solvents are similar to volatile substances used medically as anaesthetics. Glues used in model aircraft construction, and carbon tetrachloride and toluene used in dry-cleaning, have a sedative effect but are also toxic and they can damage the liver. Lighter fuel, nail polish remover, and some kinds of paint can be sniffed in order to produce dizziness and a feeling of intoxication. Hallucinations can result from continued abuse.

Chloroform and ether are of course anaesthetics and if inhaled are likely to produce unconsciousness.

Medicines containing sedatives

Medicines containing *sedatives* come mostly under the heading of cough mixtures. Many cough mixtures contain such drugs as derivatives of morphine, and because they don't only suppress coughs but sedate and give a sense of well-being, they are quite often abused: Collis Brownes, Gees Linctus and Pholcomed, for example.

Antihistamines also have a sedative effect and may be abused for this purpose.

Opiates

Finally we come to the *opiates*, the derivatives of opium, all of which are listed as Class A drugs under the 1971 Act. The most important opiate of dependence in Britain is heroin, which is diamorphine. Pethidine addicts may sometimes be encountered.

In addition to analgesic-sedative-euphoric derivatives of opium such as heroin, morphine and Pethidine, there are now synthetic opiates of which the most commonly abused is methadone, commonly called Physeptone in Britain: and Fortral and Romilar.

The opiates do, of course, have a medical use in controlling severe pain, e.g., in terminal illnesses. The present writer once had a small injection of Pethidine after having had a frozen shoulder manipulated to tear loose all the adhesions. The anaesthetic given for the operation was of short duration. The agony of this one-sided crucifixion receded like the tide going out, leaving a sense of peaceful drowsiness, after one administration of Pethidine which was never repeated.

Pure heroin is in the form of small white tablets called 'jacks', similar to saccharine tablets. It is dissolved in water for injection, and pure distilled water should be, but usually isn't, used. Heroin bought on the black market may be tablet or powder and the very impure type known as Chinese heroin looks like very fine brown sugar. Heroin from Iran is even darker, which is why it is known as 'brown belt' heroin. Supplies now come not only from the 'Golden Triangle' where Thailand, Burma and China meet, but also from Afghanistan and Pakistan.

Most heroin abusers 'fix', i.e. inject, but recently there has been an increase in the smoking of heroin, especially amongst school-children. Those who 'fix' use a tourniquet to make the vein stand out and then inject the solution with a syringe. Many get infections by using blunt and dirty needles.

Though the unaccustomed user, or the regular user taking a much larger dose than he or she is accustomed to, may suffer nausea and vomiting, and there have been many deaths by inhalation of vomit, the normal experience of the regular user of heroin is a drowsy feeling of well-being and a quasi-sexual feeling of bliss, which is greatly desired and forms the psychological dependence. Physical dependence is, however, even more important: users of heroin dread the pains of withdrawal, and find it almost impossible to reduce the dose when their inclination is to increase it to obtain the same effect as when they first began. A few hours after each 'fix', pains of withdrawal begin and increase for several hours. It may take as much as a week for them to die down if there is no further injection. Muscle cramps, perspiration, gooseflesh, sniffles, yawning, twitching and diarrhoea combined with restlessness and anxiety make the withdrawal symptoms very disagreeable indeed. It is too much to expect that a person dependent on heroin will give it up and suffer all these difficulties together with the deprivation of an extreme pleasure, without any encouragement, emotional support and medication. The addicts who have been helped to wean themselves from heroin have mostly had the withdrawal symptoms reduced to bearable proportions by the substitution of physeptone or some other sedation. Physeptone, which normally comes already dissolved in ampoule form, is itself an opiate but, as stated above, it is synthetic. It is itself addictive, but the basis of treatment in the Treatment Centres is that the withdrawal symptoms are less intolerable than those of heroin, so if physeptone is gradually substituted for heroin, the physeptone by injection can then be replaced by a physeptone linctus taken orally. Many dependents find difficulty at this stage, because the act of 'fixing' is itself part of the addiction, which will seem strange to those of us who dislike having injections at all.

Heroin dependents, who are known as 'junkies', have a low expectation of life, partly because of the danger of overdoses, hepatitis and infections, and partly because of their generally unhealthy way of life. They are often homeless and inadequately clothed and fed: everything revolves around securing their next fix, and few can afford to maintain a heroin habit on the black market without resorting to crime or prostitution. The junky is extremely unlikely to be able to hold down a job sufficiently well paid to buy heroin on the black market. Nobody who has been closely associated with a junky will envy him the allegedly better-than-orgasmic pleasure which is bought at such a terrible cost.

One addict who eventually cured himself (and mentions that most of his junkie pals are now dead) said his 'fixes' gave him a warm, comforting buzz, calmed all nasty emotions, removed the need for love, and rendered sex unnecessary. But he daily experienced withdrawal, with jangling nerves, crying, laughing, enraged, suffering stomach cramps and vomiting green bile. Another wrote that it gave more kick than cannabis and was cheaper, about the same as six pints of beer.

In the Sixties, heroin addiction caused such a scare that government Treatment Centres were set up, but the number of addicts continued to rise. In 1979 the Standing Conference on Drug Abuse warned of an approaching heroin 'epidemic' and by 1984 the word had become appropriate, with the problem spreading to schools and universities and to people in every walk of life from council estate dwellers to those in the stockbroker belt and other professional class habitats. It is impossible to know precisely how many youngsters and older people are affected, but it cannot now be fewer than a six-figure number.

Junkies present such a serious problem that Samaritans are tempted to seek a quick and easy solution.

This temptation must be resisted. Not only is it totally against the principles of The Samaritans to try to change the habits of another person without his or her consent, but it is also bound to be a source of frustration and eventually disillusionment to have the motivation for so difficult a task as giving up a drug of dependence inside a different person from the one who is dependent on the drug and has little or no motivation.

How Samaritans can help

We Samaritans have learnt to be realistic and to recognise that the majority of those who are dependent on drugs are either psychopathic or inadequate personalities bordering on the psychopathic, and in any case weak and self-indulgent characters who are incapable, even with encouragement and support, of the effort and sacrifice needed in order to be freed from dependence on a drug which they do find it possible to obtain. Only a minority who have got hooked have within themselves a strong desire to be liberated from their dependence. This minority is as worthy of the enormous amount of time and energy and patience involved as the majority is totally unworthy because their nature and character would make it certain that the effort would be totally wasted. Furthermore, the fact of attempting the impossible with the psychopathic drug abuser creates a relationship which the latter will not be slow to exploit, so that the foolishly sentimental volunteer is likely to end an unproductive involvement with the knowledge that he/she was merely facilitating the continuation of the drug dependence.

There are few things which 'sort out the men from the boys and the women from the girls' in Samaritan circles better than contact with the emotionally immature and egocentric or demanding and manipulative, of whom it must be asked if they are allegedly *not* dependent on drugs, why aren't they? Those who, in Oscar Wilde's words, 'can resist anything except temptation', are sure to be offered drugs on the streets of our big cities, and may be expected to use them if they can afford them.

A drug-dependent client of The Samaritans is a person who provides an excellent test of our principles. His or her situation will present a great temptation to the volunteer to do the forbidden thing, namely to 'solve the problem', with or without the client's consent. The desire to *do* something is understandable, but it must be restrained. The inclination to change the way of life of the client to one which would be more acceptable to the volunteer betrays the presence of a non-Samaritan in the organisation. The drug-dependent client is pre-eminently a case for befriending, which will only lead on to counselling and/or treatment if the client very much wishes this.

The listening, acceptance and concern which are included in the befriending relationship will not only establish the facts and create good rapport in those cases where a request for definite help may in due course be made, but will also assist those who do not really wish to be helped to face the reality of their situation in a way that may bear fruit at some later stage in their lives. At worst, the volunteer will avoid wasting time and energy and ending with the frustrating feeling of having been conned.

Endless patience and tolerance will be required of the volunteer in those cases where there is a genuine desire on the part of the drug dependent person to end his or her dependence. A volunteer should not be left alone with such a situation, but should work under the guidance and with the support and encouragement of a colleague. The 'enemy' may be not only the drug of abuse, but also the subculture in which it is found and which may form the environment of the drug abuser, particularly if a youngster who has come to a big town from the country. Junkies, in particular, have their own fraternity and thus minister to the drug dependent's desire to 'belong'. The junky freemasonry is so strong that any junky who appears to be escaping from it is the object of sustained attempts to win him or her back, even to the point of *giving*, freely, expensive drugs to those who have just completed a 'cure'. The Samaritans have to be seen as a group of friends who have no axe to grind and nothing to 'sell', who are befriending the drug-dependent person out of pure beneficence, and compare very favourably with the subculture in which the drug-dependent person became dependent.

Counselling and psychotherapy are beyond the scope of this essay, and as for treatment, the safest thing is to get in touch with the person's family doctor in any country where family doctors are usual. Not all countries have Treatment Centres like those in Britain, where classified drugs may be prescribed free of charge in a course of gradually diminishing dosage. The aim of the Treatment Centre is to make it unnecessary for the drug-dependent person to purchase illegal supplies, but to stick to their prescribed and gradually diminishing dose. There are areas in Britain where there are no Treatment Centres at all, in which case it is to be hoped that the Branch can obtain help from a local psychiatrist or from the casualty department of the local hospital. In extreme cases, in-patient treatment may be obtainable.

Once off the drug, the person will have to face whatever it was that caused him or her to take up the drug in the first place. Rehabilitation may be very difficult if the client cannot get a place in one of the hostels specially for this and cannot get out-patient treatment at a hospital regularly.

It has not been possible to mention more than a small proportion of the medicaments Samaritans may encounter, but every Branch should have a copy of *The British National Formulary*, which lists drugs under their chemical and proprietary names and tells what they are for and other useful information. In addition there is 'MIMS', the monthly index of medical specialities, which the Branch could obtain through a friendly GP.

Although the proportion of drug-dependent clients whom The Samaritans are able to help effectively is very small, it has added up over the years to quite a crowd of people, all of whom must be included as having been saved from a form of slow and unadmitted suicide.

Other sources of help, all of them in London but with information about other places, are: RELEASE (which has a 24-hour emergency/telephone service on 01-603 8654), 169 Commercial Street, London E1 6BW (tel. 01-377 5905);

Standing Conference on Drug Abuse (SCODA), 1–4 Hatton Place, Hatton Gardens, London EC1 (not for telephoning); Narcotics Anonymous, PO Box 246, London SW10 (tel. 01-871 0505). There is a self-help group for addicts' relatives called Families Anonymous, 88 Caledonian Road, London N1 9DN (tel. 01-278 8805).

He felt the enormous relief of speaking without prudence to someone who, he believed, understood him. The eyes seemed to offer complete friendship, the smile encouraged him to lay down for a short time the burden of secrecy.

from *The Human Factor*, GRAHAM GREENE

Befriending sex-callers – ROSEMARY HANSON

In 1973 the Central London Branch initiated a system devised by Chad to cope with the increasing number of sexually-demanding calls. This has become known as the Brenda System. Before Brenda befriending was introduced, every female volunteer coped as best she could with dozens of those calls which more often or not start with 'What colour are your knickers?' We had a situation something like this:

Volunteer answers phone.

CALLER: Have you got big tits?

VOL.: Well, . . . er . . . about average I suppose . . . Why do you want to know?

CALLER: What colour bra have you got on?

VOL.: Well, what colour do you like?

CALLER: Aren't you going to help me? (*pause*) I like nice big tits in a black lace bra. Do you wear see-through blouses?

VOL.: My name's Susan – what's yours? (*pause*) I think we've spoken before, haven't we?

Client hangs up abruptly.

The volunteer usually felt she had made no rapport with the man; she recognised him as a regular caller using different names and could not help feeling disillusioned because whatever she did to try and help she knew he would soon be back on the line claiming he had never rung before. In addition some volunteers were clearly thought to be what might be described as a softer touch than others, and callers might ring for hours on end, blocking emergency lines, in an effort to get the volunteer they desired.

Under the Brenda system all callers wanting someone to be

with them on the phone whilst they masturbate are referred to a small group of female volunteers who, for the sake of simplicity, are all known as Brenda, and are on duty at specific times especially to take such calls. Because they are a small group and they write very detailed reports after each conversation they soon get to know regular callers and can identify those who are using different names and stories, and the callers get a uniform response. In some circumstances they are willing to listen while a client masturbates, as part of a real befriending relationship.

After Brenda started, the immediate benefit was that at least we knew *who* was calling – in fact we often found that Brian, John, Peter and Bill were the same person, so the number of callers dropped quite dramatically. Since then other branches have found the same. We frequently found that callers who at first seemed *un*helpable (rather like the one in the above example), after ringing for some time, because they got a uniform response, suddenly became helpable, revealing all sorts of serious problems. Another benefit was that volunteers who had felt they were not dealing very well with these callers felt relieved and in general the Branch seemed to feel that we were trying in an organised way to help callers who had been blocking the lines unprofitably.

I know many people feel that the Samaritans, a crisis organisation, should not waste time trying to befriend sex-callers. There is no doubt that amongst those making sex-calls is quite a high percentage of manipulative and disturbed men. Chad's original contention was that there are also men who, although they approach us in the same way, have problems which cause them intense distress and who are ready to accept our help, if we can manage to make the initial rapport with them. This has proved to be true: we have found that a surprisingly high number of sex-callers are depressed and suicidal.

In some cases the sex-caller's first aggressive approach may be rather like the giggles of a group of children in a phone-box – a testing of our shockability and understanding. A call which exemplifies this started with abusive and crude sexual language, but after some minutes of the volunteer meeting this with calm understanding, the caller called out to someone, 'It's all right, I think they'll talk to you OK,' and handed over the phone to his fourteen-year-old girlfriend who was pregnant.

Each time Brenda talks to a new client she tries to assess whether the caller wants or would accept a real befriending relationship; our aim is to help the client stop making what are usually called obscene calls. We usually have in our minds the following questions:

1. Why does he need to masturbate on the phone?
2. What happens when he does it privately? Is there something physically wrong? Is he worried that his penis is too big or too small?
3. Does *he* see it as a problem?
4. Has he ever had sex? Was it a happy experience?
5. What are his relationships like – with family, friends, work-mates, girlfriend/wife?
6. Does he feel unhappy, guilty, isolated, depressed?
7. Is he suicidal?

Above all we are honest about what we can and can't offer. It is obviously to our advantage as well as his that he should not imagine that he can talk us into anything or claim that there has been a misunderstanding because we were too shy to be frank or suppose that any of us will take a different line from the one we have all agreed. It is crucial to the Brenda system that each caller should be identified and a policy agreed on by all the Brendas and communicated to the caller so that he may discuss it and, we hope, accept it as reasonable and co-operate with it.

We have found that our honesty induces an honest response from the caller, and that though many are very demanding at first, they become undemanding once they have the security of knowing they can ring and knowing what will happen when they do. Somehow the masturbation part becomes gradually less important once it has been accepted.

What we do *not* offer, and never have, is a kind of dial-a-wank service, with all female volunteers listening to all masturbating callers in the hope of making rapport with someone who is almost certain to hang up once he has ejaculated but will probably be back on the line before long wanting to do it again. Apart from the odd psychopath who uses a sexual rather than their usual aggressive-manipulative approach, the sex-callers, especially if they have a long history of making random calls, are prone to guilt and shame, so dial-a-wank has little to be said in its favour if it leaves the volunteer feeling used and useless, and the caller despising himself yet knowing he'll do it again when the urge comes. The kinder the volunteer, the more ashamed the caller may be, the moment the tension has been relieved. Because they feel they have treated someone badly who was trying to help them, they hate themselves for conning her into it. They want to forget about it as quickly as possible – until the next crisis of frustration, when they will use another identity. And so the pattern continues, with *us* inadvertently reinforcing the client's own low opinion of himself. Our refusing to 'help' without first having made a rapport and discovered the cause of his needing to masturbate on the phone is bad luck on those rare clients for whom 'Just this once . . .' might have been right, but we are trying to break a pattern of behaviour.

I think it is possible to turn something negative into something positive. As Chad Varah explains in his book *Telephone Masturbators and the Brenda System for befriending them*, befriending a caller while he masturbates can be beneficial, leading him to revise his opinion both of himself and of women. But what if the client becomes hooked on Brenda, swapping one addiction for another? Several times in the early days of this system we rather nervously broached this subject with a client, only to find him relieved to discuss it and agreeing that he would limit his wanking calls (usually setting a target of so many days between them), while feeling free to ring us to discuss how things are going in between them. As usual we get steamed up about things which clients solve for themselves! However, we have noticed with certain types of callers – usually married and with good jobs, perhaps their own business (*not* people who are socially isolated) that a domestic crisis or extra pressure at work can trigger off renewed frenetic wanking activity. When this does happen, if we are clever, it can be used to give the client new insight into the cause of the problem.

There are certainly a number of callers who are considered by volunteers to be unhelpable, at least by us. They include quite a number of unemployed young men. For them making these calls seems almost to be a way of filling time. They are generally dispirited and bored; they complain that they cannot afford to go out much, although when they do they have no difficulty in meeting and getting on with girls. We think it is important to discourage them from getting addicted. A similar pattern has emerged among shift workers – single men whose social lives are non-existent because they work nights, and married men who get home several hours before their wives and children.

How do you make that initial rapport which persuades the client to stay on the line even though you won't talk about the colour of your knickers? Answering questions about your underwear or vital statistics with 'Why do you want to know?' is usually counter-productive – it starts us on a childish conversational ball-game with each side refusing to give way. Both sides know why, so neither is being honest. It is the sort of question which, if the client does answer, does not progress the conversation any further and it tells you little about him as a person. If a volunteer answers in a light-hearted vein this too can result in stalemate, and may be interpreted by the client as reinforcing the view he has of women – they laugh at him. However aggressive the client may sound, he is quite likely to be frightened of women. And however cool the volunteer tries to be she may respond to his aggression by being defensive; it is natural to be nervous of being pushed into saying things you do not want to say, however sympathetic you are.

It helps to bear in mind that you cannot be physically attacked on the telephone, and that you don't *have* to answer questions – you can take control of the conversation by asking questions yourself – and if they are the right questions you will show the client that you understand how he is feeling and are sorry about it and may surprise him into responding positively. So, one response might be 'You must be feeling very frustrated – do you often feel like this – it must be terrible. Has something gone wrong in your sex-life?' This might lead you to discover he has no sex-life – cannot make a relationship with women – never has had a girlfriend – he is frightened his penis is too big or too small – he has been laughed at when he tried to make love – or he is married and sex with his wife is not good – already you are befriending the client. You haven't blocked the conversation by *saying* 'I am not going to discuss my underwear', although in fact you are not going to.

If the caller starts with 'Have you got big tits?' – a fairly standard opener – you might reply 'Is that what you like? Have you ever had sex with a girl with big tits?' – showing that you're prepared to talk about the subject. You may discover that he never has – is very isolated indeed – or used to have a relationship but she left or died and life has never been the same since . . .

Brendas are not permitted to answer questions about their own sexual experience, but if any of them feel a bit feeble saying 'it's against the rules', it seems perfectly acceptable to me to tell a client that discussing your own sex-life makes you feel uncomfortable; if you do it kindly your honesty may open up the conversation. You may find out if the client wants to make you feel bad or wants you to make him feel better – Chad's criterion, and a very useful guide to which sex-callers we can help.

If, in spite of all our friendly but firm understanding and sympathy, the client hangs up on us this does not necessarily mean a failure. He will probably ring again, hoping to find a softer touch, but again he will be referred to Brenda. The uniform response seems to make callers reflect. Admittedly some disappear and probably ring other branches. Some come back even after weeks or months and decide to accept what we offer. This happened with a young client of ours who seemed particularly cut-off and isolated and unbelievably ignorant about sex. It eventually turned out that he was disabled and did indeed lead a very impoverished life. He lived alone with his elderly father; he had no privacy and no experience on which to base his fantasies. He is befriended now by a male volunteer and only rings occasionally, usually just for a chat.

When we recognise clients using different names we can gently suggest that they stick to one name and they are often relieved that they don't have to lie and try to manipulate us. With those clients who ring to tell and retell a fantasy under the pretext that these bizarre events are true and a great worry to them, it is the uniform response which breaks through to the problem behind this need. The whole system would break down if any one Brenda was manipulable and failed to stick to the policies agreed.

One of the things we have learnt is that very few of our callers have *only* a sexual problem. Many are severely depressed or suffering from a variety of personality disorders – the sex-call is the presenting problem, a rather muffled cry for help. It is easy to understand that some sexual problems can cause a reactive depression. If, for example, you love your wife or girlfriend but have been impotent for some months, you are likely to become depressed by this.

A caller whose story illustrates this is Harry, a married man who had been impotent for some years. He eventually went to his doctor but, too nervous to be explicit, simply said 'I'm having trouble in bed.' Unfortunately the doctor prescribed sleeping pills, which he later took all at once, but was found and resuscitated. Although he started as a typical 'Have you got big tits?' caller it was clear quite quickly that he was depressed. It took several years to discover why; unexpectedly he came in one day and some time later agreed to see another doctor. It seems likely that pills he was taking for epilepsy were causing the impotence which in turn caused depression.

It is perhaps less easy to understand that sexual problems, including the sex-call itself, can be actual symptoms of depression. Depression can cause impotence or an inability to climax. In addition, failure in a sexual context can lead to anxiety which can lead to another failure. Frustration builds up and intensifies the depression, and can lead to suicidal feelings and eventually to parasuicide or suicide.

A good example is Ben, an engineer who had a severe breakdown after a divorce. We did not of course know that this was his situation when he started ringing. He used to make sex-calls to us and to others. But it seemed to us that beneath the aggression was a lack of confidence. After three years of Brenda befriending, I am happy to say he has a girl friend and is much happier. Three years is a long time, but like so many of these callers, Ben needed patience and understanding.

Depression affects sexual performance without taking away the physical frustration. The listlessness and lack of energy which characterise the illness of depression make it impossible for most depressed men to do anything positive about their frustration. Depression often robs the sufferer of the imagination needed to fantasise. Another symptom of severe depression is an inability to communicate, which is liable to increase until the sufferer is completely cut-off and isolated – certainly in no state to make new relationships or improve old ones. Like so many of our depressed clients they may be unaware that they are ill and ignorant of the correlation between sexual malfunction and depression. They may have identified their sex-problem as the cause, not the symptom, of the trouble.

This was the case with a client called Pete. He rang intending to make a sex-call. He sounded very sad and depressed. He said he had tried to have sex with a girl recently and hadn't been able to get an erection. She had not been very understanding. Now he was worried that he was impotent, and also that the girl would tell mutual friends in the pub. After several long conversations it turned out that this young man had been very happily married and then his wife, after giving birth to the baby they both wanted very much, had died of kidney failure 5 years previously. He had never had a chance to mourn properly; he was encouraged by friends and relatives to 'start a new life' before getting over the tragedy. He became very cut-off and isolated. He knew he should go out more, and it was at this point that he started going to the pub and met this girl. But he was in no state to make a new relationship.

Clients sometimes say that they make sexually demanding calls because they cannot get an erection on their own, that to pick up a phone is much easier than picking up a girl, and that to masturbate while listening to a strange woman's voice involves the least energy and commitment on their part. The same client may speak in a low, flat tone, answer in monosyllables, seem lacking in imagination and be curiously apathetic even when obviously masturbating – this is something we often notice. He may express the wish that he could sublimate all sexual desire, seeing it as the cause of unhappiness and distress – 'I wish I could cut it off . . .' If he has not had a girlfriend for some time, or never, does not go out much, has few or no friends to go out with, no hobbies or interests, no job or no interest in his job, the volunteer would do well to ask about his sleeping, eating and concentration and to find out if he feels life is worth living – he may be very suicidal indeed.

Exposers ('flashers') are unlikely to be Brenda callers – the point about their particular obsession is that they need to be seen and not heard – but many are tempted to come in and flash because they know we will not report them. If this does happen we usually say we will leave the room for a few minutes to make a tactful cup of tea. Wanking in the centre can precipitate distressing scenes with the client rushing out in tears, overcome with guilt, and the volunteer very upset because she has made him worse not better. The problem is that the client, even if he did not intend to flash, is unable to 'control himself' and we have little or no warning that this is about to happen (although a number of volunteers have said that they have noticed an expression on a client's face just before flashing that can only be described as childish which could be a signal). In many cases fear of being caught and the public humiliation of prosecution is no deterrent: simply the cause of appalling anguish *after* exposing. Many of our clients have said that something 'takes over', something which however hard they try to resist, they cannot, even though they know on a rational level it is self-destructive. The most we can say about the many exposers who have been to us is that we have kept a few out of prison and have been instrumental in getting a few to accept professional help. It is rare in our experience that they will accept befriending by a male volunteer.

While exposers are often eager to visit our centre (albeit briefly), sex-callers are usually hesitant to do so. Some people believe that if a sex-caller is serious about wanting help he must be prepared to come in. This is a lot to expect *before* rapport has been established. I think we should not underestimate the fear these clients may feel at the prospect of a confrontation. Many have never made any kind of relationship with a woman, or indeed a man, before, and although *we* may be convinced that face-to-face befriending could help them it is not easy to sell the idea to a man who is chronically shy and embarrassed.

Over the years we have come to feel that two things are most important in the administration of a Brenda system. First, if you are going to refer a client to someone 'special' he must not be made to feel rejected. It is vital that the whole branch is trained how to make such referrals in a 'Samaritan' way, and one which encourages the caller to ring back if necessary. Everyone must be very clear about whom to refer. All too easily Brenda can be used as a resident 'expert' to turn to when a volunteer feels out of his or her depth – thus the poor man whose marriage is on the rocks because his wife has just discovered he is a transvestite, or the frightened boy who thinks he has VD could be erroneously referred to Brenda. Secondly, we think that Brendas should be selected because listening to a man masturbate (and we think this should not entail giving personal statistics, details of your own sex life, or acting out the client's fantasies) is just part of the compassion they feel for the client; they should be neither overly keen nor disapproving. Most Brenda volunteers say they find it rewarding because they get to know clients well and can see at least some of them change gradually, sometimes frustratingly slowly, into happier people. They will need a lot of support from other volunteers. We have found that Brenda duties are taxing, not so much because of the subject of the calls but because of the more directive, assessing role we find ourselves in. Although this is not easy, essentially it is still a Samaritan role.

When we first started we were anxious about our lack of 'expertise' in the field, and when we consulted experts and they told us we probably knew more about telephone masturbators than they did, this was scarcely reassuring. In fact perhaps the most important thing we have learnt is that it is not expertise that our clients want, but befriending.

To sum up: Brendas now *know* that their system can help a good many callers whom no one else could help, and that the proportion of their callers who were right to turn to The Samaritans is at least as great as in other categories. Brenda is essentially a befriender, even though she has to be more directive sometimes than other Samaritans, and the relationship she establishes with her callers is a befriending relationship, never a sexual one. She herself is not turned on by her work, but is often moved almost to tears, and quite often bored with the same old tales. Her case conferences, with nearly 100% present, produce a sensible and practical policy for each caller, and Brendas are loyal to one another in sticking to it. Maybe other types of persistent callers could be helped more if similar care was taken to work as a team.

It is a sad thing that in the British Isles the number of Branches operating a Brenda system has declined, and sadder still that some have been tempted to excuse this by alleging that it had been found not to work. We know that where it is operated in the way I have described, it cannot fail to work, unless non-Brenda volunteers are either failing to pass sexually-demanding callers on to Brenda, or are hanging up on them, or are undermining Brenda's work by sharing fantasies with masturbating callers.

One thing is certain: the sexually-demanding caller will not stop ringing simply because a Branch wishes he would give up, and rebuffs him. If a Branch is sufficiently rude and rejecting, it may offload the problem onto nearby Branches. Or even distant Branches – Central London has had a lot of calls from the USA since most US Branches felt they were getting swamped with Brenda calls and determined to stamp them out. Perhaps now that there are dozens of call girls offering to share fantasies at a price (charged by credit card), they will find it easier to respond to the sexually-demanding callers whom this does not help, because what they really need is befriending.

The language of friendship is not words but meanings.

HENRI DAVID THOREAU

Aid on AIDS – CHAD VARAH

There's a virus called HTLV III. It's fragile, and dies quickly outside the body. You can't catch it by shaking hands, hugging, ordinary kissing or using the same mug or loo as an infected person. It's doubtful whether you can catch it by 'wet' kissing: it doesn't seem to be spread by saliva, but it is by blood, semen and faeces. It's impossible to get it from the chalice at Holy Communion. You *can* get it from sex with an infected person, vaginally, anally, or orally; or by the blood of an infected person (e.g. sharing needles with a drug addict).

If you get the virus, your body will make 'antibodies' against it, but this can take three months, or even more. Tests can show these antibodies, but the infected person can pass on the virus before this. Some people with the HTLV III virus contract AIDS (Acquired Immune Deficiency Syndrome). Others don't, but can still pass the virus on.

There isn't a disease called 'Aids'. People who die as a result of AIDS die of all sorts of illnesses, of the lungs, skin, intestines or brain. AIDS has destroyed the body's defences against them.

If you have a test which proves positive, you are not likely to get AIDS, but you could pass the virus on, so be responsible. Don't tell anyone except a Samaritan, or the Terrence Higgins Trust, BM AIDS, London WC1N 3XX. Their Helpline is 01-833 2971.

It seems that after two years 75 out of a typical 100 men with antibodies were well, 15 had minor illnesses caused by HLTV III, and 10 had AIDS of whom 4 died.

Incest – CHAD VARAH

Everyone knows that incest is wrong, and that even when it does not include the sexual abuse of children, the effects are likely to be damaging, especially to any on whom it was inflicted against their will. But Samaritans have to realise that saying this does nothing to solve the problem or lead those involved in it to turn to them. Indeed, as in the case of suicide itself, mere denunciation reduces the chances of our being allowed to limit the distress and damage caused.

Incest is now following homosexuality and suicide as a formerly taboo subject which is beginning to be brought into the open, with a similar result: there is more of it than was previously suspected.

We must distinguish between the taboo against committing incest, i.e. having sexual intercourse with close relatives, which is a valuable protection that society must not lose, and the taboo against discussing the subject, the ending of which is likely in time to reduce the incidence of incest. Indeed, the conspiracy of silence has prevented many unwilling participants in incest from seeking help. Children especially, when subjected to incestuous intercourse or other sexual abuse, are usually sworn to secrecy by their molester, or are told that if they complained about such an unthinkable act no one would believe them, for who ever heard any talk of such things? The child almost certainly feels shame about the whole matter, and may also experience irrational guilt, as though she (or he) were the guilty party.

It is, sadly, true that very often a child's complaint will not be believed, sometimes because the child's mother or other adult does not want to believe it. Courts require corroborative evidence of a kind which in the nature of the offence is hardly ever available, and suggestions that England should adopt the methods pioneered in Texas are resisted on the ground that dreadful miscarriages of justice may occur if children's fantasies are accepted as facts, or if it is supposed that they could never persist in malicious lies. In Texas, sexually-abused children may be questioned as to what exactly happened by child psychologists using male and female dolls, and the videotape of the interview is used in Court, which avoids having a timid child bullied and browbeaten by an intimidating lawyer who cares nothing for truth or justice and is concerned only to get his client off.

Societies for helping the child victims of sexual abuse always emphasise that there should be *no secrets*, no agreement to keep something from the child's parents, and the same rule would be invaluable in cases of incest at any age where one of the parties is, or has gradually become, an unwilling victim.

To understand why incest is as prevalent as it now appears to be, it is necessary to examine the sexual attitudes of the one who almost always takes the initiative, the male. Almost all incest in western societies is father-daughter, brother-sister, uncle-niece, grandfather-granddaughter, and it may involve either rape, near-rape (i.e. determined, sustained and repeated demands for compliance) or seduction. In seduction intended to lead to intercourse, the male almost invariably takes the initiative; where young girls behave seductively, as they sometimes do in order to get attention, they are not seeking intercourse and may be horrified to discover what a monster they have aroused.

Mother-son incest, with the mother taking the initiative, seems to be widespread only in Japan, though it is alleged to be increasing in one-parent families in the USA. Japan also has the male-initiated incest found in other countries.

The key

The key to understanding incest is the fact that the human male is spontaneously sexed, is very easily aroused (unless thoroughly absorbed in something else), and when aroused is aware of it and impatient for sexual gratification. It is no use blaming the male for this: his physiology is essential to the reproduction of the species; but it is meant to be within the restraints of moral scruples and social conventions, without which he would, like many animals, copulate with any female he fancied and could subdue, if not prevented by stronger and possessive males.

Human beings are capable of romantic love, of tenderness, of faithfulness. But the rampant male animal is not abolished by this veneer of civilisation, only inhibited. If alone and unobserved, for instance, he will masturbate whenever he feels the urge, unless he has been terrorised or conditioned against this useful outlet. His favourite fantasies may well include being in a secluded place with one or more women who are tied up or otherwise at his mercy.

The pituitary gland leads the testes to produce a regular supply of the hormone testosterone, which causes sexual aggression. The female produces a little of this hormone, and is capable of *some* sexual spontaneity (and indeed masturbates, though not as universally or frequently as the male), but on the whole she is responsively sexed and does not often experience explicitly sexual desires unless provoked to these.

With this picture of the male in mind, it is easy to see that the intimacies of family life may furnish occasions where the male sees something he finds arousing without the female concerned being aware of the effect she is having. Even within the family, females normally behave with a certain modesty or shyness, but this is mostly in deference to their own feelings and not out of fear of the effect of glimpses of femininity on the males of the household, which they tend to underestimate. There is a happy medium: exaggerated care may have as disturbing an effect as too great laxity.

In most families the incest taboo, plus the operation of the truism 'familiarity breeds contempt', leads the males to find the forbidden females in the household uninteresting sexually. This particularly applies to siblings: other chaps' sisters are strange and exciting, one's own are 'old hat' and boring – God knows why they're forbidden for who could want them! Philip Roth, in *Portnoy's Complaint*, tells how his hero locks himself in the bathroom, finds bra and panties worn by his sister in the laundry basket, strings them up as if they were on a girl, and masturbates at them; but this does not prove that he lusts after his sister. He is using the bra and panties as a symbol of the female. A pornographic photograph would have been much more effective.

Father-daughter attractions differ from those of brother-sister in that a man looking at his daughter may see a representation of his wife at the age at which he fell in love with her, and if the sexual relationship with his wife has deteriorated he may find the youthful appeal of his daughter very powerful. But in the vast majority of such cases he is truly loving and does nothing about it because he feels it would be wrong and because he does not want to damage either her sexual future or the relation of affection which he already has with the girl. If she is 'Daddy's girl' she is *less* likely to be at risk.

A girl's sexually-hungry older male relatives may display affection to her quite innocently, but if play leads to horseplay, including such things as wrestling and tickling, the man may find himself getting an unplanned erection. He should, of course, immediately desist and cool down, but if he doesn't, he may wish to pursue the matter and may manage to get the girl excited without her understanding what is happening. After a series of such skirmishes he may be able to take advantage of her sexually.

Where quite small children are concerned, there are often deep-seated psychological reasons for sexual interference with them, but even without these a little girl at play, with legs unselfconsciously spread wide, may serve as a sort of symbol of female sexuality in much the same way as Portnoy's sister's bra and panties, but at the same time being warm living flesh. For most of us, of course, the symbol would be either unrecognised or ineffective: the child is simply too small to be of any sexual use and, quite apart from protective feelings, it wouldn't occur or wouldn't appeal to a normal man to follow it up in any way. Even if the child exhibited her immature vulva and the word 'cunt' came into the man's mind, any further thoughts would be of penetrable adult genitals surrounded by pubic hair and capable during coition of giving pleasure to their owners.

Nearly all men are in some sense open to sexual interest nearly all the time. But except for a few who are disposed to incest, and another few who would not have planned it but fell into it through weakness when an unexpected opportunity occurred, they exclude from their calculations near relatives, girls under 16, and the wives or girlfriends of their brothers or best friends.

Deterrents

Deterrents to incest are inward and outward. Inwardly, the conscience should say 'this would be wrong' even if the instinct does not say 'this is sick, it's off-putting'. Outwardly, society does not tolerate incest and punishes it, often severely. If it is rape rather than seduction, the victim may be impossible to silence except by killing her, and it is only the psychopathic who don't look far enough ahead to see that, and would not care if they did. Many of those who commit rape, whether incestuous or not, *are* psychopathic, incapable of love or conscience, without prudence, and determined to have what they want when they want it, regardless.

A lot depends on the nature of the family in which incest is either contemplated or has already occurred. In a respectable family, exposure of the act to the other members of the family, even if there is no question of the police being involved, would be such an embarrassment as to prevent it if it hadn't yet occurred or to punish it if it had.

There are, of course, a number of precautions that can be taken to make incest less likely to occur. An obvious one is the provision of sleeping arrangements which protect girls from being too easily get-at-able, and care in avoiding them being alone in the house regularly or for long periods. Yet they must not be made nervous, nor must the male members of the family be made to feel they are under suspicion when there is no justification for this. A carefree attitude should be felt and imparted by the mother, who may even feel that her family is sufficiently open and outgoing for nudity to be practised without anxiety. (It is well known that constant exposure to nudity is anaphrodisiac – in nudist colonies, scanty garments are rightly regarded as more provocative. This does not deny the powerful aphrodisiac effect of occasional or unexpected nakedness.)

Secondly, there must be open discussion in the family of all sorts of sexual problems such as are likely to arise out of the news, and this will probably include the subject of incest.

Everyone should be clear that family relationships are precious and unique and essential to the relaxed life of a happy family. Confusion would be caused if any members were sexual objects to others.

Thirdly, the mother, who is the responsible *female* adult, is well advised to be quietly aware of what the males are up to. She obviously has an interest in her husband being content; she does not want him sexually deprived and restless if she can help it. She should also encourage the love-life of her sons and welcome their girlfriends to the family home. But whatever defences the woman provides, we must remember that it is the man who may make her prudence necessary.

Even now that it is surfacing more, incest is not apparently so widespread that the possibility of it should be allowed to have a destructive effect on the life of an ordinary family. Indeed, the wise precautions against incest are also to some extent precautions against rape by strangers, and should help to make the family more carefree.

Some families are more at risk than others, though it must not be assumed that such families are always at risk. First we must put families where the man is alcoholic. Alcohol reduces inhibitions, and drunkenness is used as an excuse for many transgressions, and this 'I wasn't myself' or 'I didn't know what I was doing' diminishes guilt.

One-parent families, and families where the mother has a succession of live-in boyfriends, are more at risk, as are those where the mother is severely handicapped.

Collusion

We rightly think of incest as a matter where the male is the villain of the piece, and some women are afraid that this fact will be obscured if they permit the subject of collusion to be discussed. I am not speaking of female consent to incestuous acts committed upon themselves, but of the fact that some women collude in the incestuous use of their daughter by their husband by choosing not to know or believe that it is going on, because of preferring its continuance to the destructive effect of a showdown or the scandal and financial loss resulting from exposure and police prosecution. One can only pity the girl whose own mother will not believe or protect her, but one must not be utterly without compassion for the woman who is terrified of the probable consequences of her accusing and obstructing her husband. Those whose immediate response on discovering a case of incest is to insist on calling the police are unfit to be Samaritans, because it is the people involved who have to live with the results of this, and it is they alone who should freely make any decision about what is to be done. We Samaritans do not tell our callers what to do, according to our own desires or prejudices, and do not inform anyone outside the organisation of alleged crimes of which we hear.

This policy also protects us from making fools of ourselves when sexually-demanding callers utilise fantasies based on imaginary rape to excite themselves when making masturbating calls.

It should be noted that incest is found in all classes of society, and the higher the social standing of the family concerned, the higher the price to be paid by bringing the guilty secret into the open.

Samaritan response

Does this mean that the man who brazens it out with his wife, and says when challenged that if he is sent to prison his earnings will disappear, should be allowed to get away with it? The answer is that that is not for us to decide. It is for the family, who should be well befriended and also offered professional help if they wish it, to make a plan which will enable the family to survive as a family.

Samaritans know that problems are not solved by flying into a rage and hitting out blindly, and that people who just want to give vent to their feelings of outrage are self-indulgent and immature (like the offender!) and could never be Samaritans. We refuse to accept that trying to understand what has happened and why, and to seek the best achievable outcome, represents any sort of condoning.

As Samaritans, we have to be prepared to take calls and accept confidences from unwilling victims of incest, from partly-willing victims, from partners, from perpetrators, from colluders – in short, from any of the persons involved. The oh-how-terrible-this-must-be-stopped-at-once response is of no use to any of these categories, not even the unwilling victim.

In matters as difficult and emotive as incest, it is vital for us to remember that we are befrienders, and that what we offer is a listening therapy. We have to be calm and accepting, and give the callers a chance to understand their situation better by telling it. It is not our responsibility to solve the problem, or to punish anyone.

There are plenty of adults who cannot handle the physical and emotional intensities of sex; putting this kind of overload on to the nervous system of a child may be more than he/she can bear. The law wisely says no consent is valid before someone is old enough to understand the perils and consequences of his/her agreement. How much more strongly we feel when the older person is a mother or father, and the younger a son or daughter.

NANCY FRIDAY, *Men in Love*

Fanaticism – CHAD VARAH

The Samaritans are listeners. Whatever their human failings in the world outside, when they come on duty they leave behind their self-regard and self-concern in order to be as far as possible what the clients wish them to be, need them to be. They have to accept the caller as he is, and befriend him whilst he seeks his own way forward at his own pace. That is why Samaritans are not permitted to try to 'sell' their own views or beliefs, which would not fit the caller and in his vulnerable, suggestible state could approximate to brainwashing or at the least deter him from frankness in confiding his doubts, fears and hopes.

The implacable opposition of The Samaritans to crisis intervention services dominated by religious bodies whose members may exhort instead of respecting the caller's own philosophy does not mean that devout believers (or supporters of a political party) are barred as volunteers. A person may hold firm religious or political convictions without being a fanatic. There are some religious sects or political parties which no one but a fanatic would join, but others whose rigid beliefs are imposed only on their own members, even though they may have some fanatical adherents who wish to impose them on everybody. The Samaritans themselves have principles which are binding on members.

How does one recognise a fanatic? He feels threatened if anyone disagrees with his pronouncements, and becomes anxious if any part of his beliefs is challenged, lest the whole structure be undermined. His satisfaction in imposing his ideology on others is short-lived and needs regular renewal. He would like to be a dictator whose decrees are obeyed without question. Some fanatics have been.

The fanatic tries to embody his beliefs in legislation, so that people who do not share them may be forced to act in accordance with them, or be punished. Nothing could be more contrary to the spirit of The Samaritans.

Three subjects on which fanatics try to impede the work of The Samaritans are abortion, homosexuality and pornography, all related to human sexuality and therefore emotive. It should be clear to all Samaritans that their private attitudes to these matters and the practice of themselves and their families are their own business. But fanatical attempts to impose these attitudes on the public at large, or to mention them to callers, absolutely disqualify the person from being a Samaritan.

The caller has been offered befriending, not indoctrination or condemnation. A caller with an unwanted pregnancy must be befriended and thus calmed sufficiently to consider what she wants to do about the situation. All possibilities should be frankly discussed. When she has made her choice, whether termination or continuing to term, she must be told where she can get expert advice and help. A Samaritan whose private religious convictions are totally against abortion has no problem about keeping these private and giving the information required. Naturally, because Samaritans believe in the caller's freedom of choice, as an organisation we have to be against removal of that freedom by making one of the options unavailable.

The homosexual caller must be befriended, and thus helped to find his or her way to a fuller sexual life such as a heterosexual is free to have, without any mention being made of any religious objections the volunteer may have been taught. As an organisation we cannot but be glad that the Wolfenden Committee recommendations were passed, decriminalising homosexual acts between consenting adults in private. Similar freedom for the autoerotic client dependent on pornography for his sexual gratification, recommended by the Williams Committee, must obviously be similarly welcomed by The Samaritans as an organisation.

Our tenderness towards the clients, and our respect for their right (and indeed, duty) to make their own moral decisions, make us many enemies. Let them all be outside, in the cruel world that drives the clients to seek refuge in Samaritan befriending.

O eloquent, just and mighty Death! Whom none could advise, thou hast persuaded; what none hath dared, thou hast done; and whom all the world hath flattered, thou onelie hast cast out of the world and despised. Thou hast drawne together all the farre stretched greatnesses, all the pride, crueltie, and ambition of man, and covered it all over with these two narrow words, *Hic jacet* . . .

Unfinished History of the World, SIR WALTER RALEIGH

to be nobody but yourself in a world which is doing its best night and day to make you everybody else, is to fight the hardest battle which any human being can fight, and never stop fighting.

e. e. cummings

How can Samaritans be protected from useless manipulation by the psychopath?

— DOMINIQUE ALESSANDRI

The statement of a young volunteer after a year's experience in The Samaritans seems to be a good introduction to this question.

'I came here thinking that we ought to do everything possible to help those who ask for it – now I see clearly that there are some people for whom we can do nothing more.'

This was by no means the remark of a discouraged person – her faith and enthusiasm for the actions of The Samaritans remain undiminished. At first glance this seems to present a contradiction; yet it does not. For the Samaritan of the Gospel performed two very distinct acts:

First, he brought immediate assistance to a man in need.

Secondly, and much more importantly, he gave him the possibility of setting out again in life, freely and with dignity.

This is the story of an action which is completely exemplary: an anonymous act (the choice of a Samaritan is free of any religious or moral conviction), disinterested, efficient, and limited in time. This action in no way left the recipient dependent on the Samaritan but, on the contrary, free to return to live among other men. In addition, the action did not inconvenience the Samaritan in any way. He possessed the material means (time and money) to bring this help without neglecting his own occupations – this, too, is not without importance. And it is this special meaning of the Samaritan's help that the parable emphasises.

Two essential questions now arise that define the limits of this help.

Will the Samaritan's help have this liberating power for the person to whom it is granted, or will it be only temporarily effective, leaving the recipient in a state of dependence on his helpers and society?

Can the Samaritan's help be effective without carrying a prejudice (either moral or material) towards the organisation, which would endanger its capacity to help other clients?

In the case of people given the rough, general label of 'psychopaths', these questions have a very special relevance. Psychopaths, or 'immature personalities', comprise all categories of individuals whose emotions have remained blocked at an infantile stage. The extent of this blockage, as well as the stage at which it occurs, varies, as do their disorders and degrees of psychopathy.

If we limit ourselves to plain psychopathy, the business of enumerating, describing and classifying psychopathic disorders is of only very limited interest for Samaritans. There would even be a certain degree of danger for Samaritans in believing that one can, by reading descriptive and theoretical work, learn to 'label a client' and anticipate the surprises and dangers that he has in reserve. By so doing, The Samaritans' spontaneity – one of the most important qualities in their response – risks being weakened.

It seems infinitely more appropriate during the volunteers' training to prepare them to face these dangers when they present themselves in practice. Two distinct aspects of this topic should therefore be considered. The first would summarise the most obvious and frequent traps laid by these psychopaths, according to the characteristics of their personality. The second, and the most essential, would be to get The Samaritans to ask themselves why they fall into certain traps, and to consider both the need for and the means of avoiding them.

Certain characteristics often found in psychopaths

An enormous emotional greed: their demands for help constitute 'the proof that they are loved', but no sooner is this proof of love obtained, than it is rejected – deemed insufficient. And so their demands will be renewed. They can be materialistic (money, social aid), or emotional (a desire to monopolise attention, a desire for pity, a desire to challenge through aggressive behaviour, then see just how much they can be loved despite this). These demands and challenges can only become more and more incessant and abusive. With this 'emotional greed' is associated an incapacity to love of surprising magnitude. What they are looking for is to seduce, to attract pity, to manipulate. Other people are for them only the instruments of their desires. Aggressiveness always lies behind their demands. The more one has, in acceding to their demands, given them the hope that they can always be satisfied, the less able they are to tolerate frustration. Here we must point out a danger for Samaritans. If they allow this kind of hope to develop in a psychopath, a perilous 'return to reality' is to be feared the day they refuse to go further in befriending him. Faced with frustration, the psychopath's aggressive nature will be released, often in an impulsive and destructive manner, be it against himself (in impulsive suicide or some sort of auto-destructive act), or against a Samaritan or the entire organisation.

It seems that in most cases the psychopath is incapable of overcoming his drive or controlling his behaviour. In extreme cases, criminal acts are committed without the psychopath feeling in any way responsible. He does not know 'what came over him'!

The psychopath, in an attempt to obtain something, or in an act of revenge, will also take more elaborate measures such as various forms of blackmail, of which the most delicate – threat to commit suicide – should be noted by Samaritans. In dangling the threat of suicide, the psychopath tries simultaneously to obtain what he wants and specifically attack The Samaritans. While trying to burden them with the responsibility for his death, he will try to spread uneasiness, remorse and scandal within The Samaritans. This blackmail is sometimes followed by impulsive suicide. However, usually it concludes with a simple attempt or fake attempt. But what would one get involved in if one gave in to this blackmail? The manipulator is going to obtain what he wants, and that will defuse the conflict for the moment. But it will begin all over again, and each time for motives which become more and more frivolous. Thus one becomes involved in a particularly dangerous relationship, destined to failure. If such a case presents itself to Samaritans, it seems important, from the moment a response is to be made, to think of future consequences, after having, of course, weighed the suicidal risk.

Besides the true delinquents and criminals whom one will be dealing with among these psychopaths, there will be all sorts of 'social cases' among The Samaritans' clientele: people incapable of holding down jobs, unable to take care of a family, accumulating debts, continuously having problems with neighbours, involved in minor delinquency, alcoholics, drug addicts, sexual deviants, and so on.

The stories told by these people of their sad lot can be very upsetting for those who listen. It seems that throughout their lives disaster has followed them, they are rejected by everyone, catastrophe accumulates along their path. The Samaritans must learn to control their own feelings in response to such touching stories. They must realise that it would be unwise, out of excessive emotion, to take any decision without expert advice.

Sometimes there is a really urgent need for social aid, and this cannot, in these cases, be systematically refused.

But if one is clear-headed enough to control these emotions, impose firm limits to their demands, and not, under any circumstances, allow the assistance given to be detrimental to the needs of other clients, the risks that one takes can be greatly reduced. Furthermore, when having any dealings with a psychopath, it is of the utmost importance that The Samaritans stick together, and that all the members concerned are aware of what is acceptable and what is not, in each case. The psychopath has a particular flair for discovering even the smallest weakness in the cohesion of a group. He will *always* try to get from those in the group who seem more hesitant (in general the most inexperienced) what he has been unable to obtain from the others. If he succeeds in this, he will not only achieve his ends but, in so doing, will cause one or more Samaritans to infringe the discipline of the organisation and have to be penalised. His hope is thus to stir up trouble within the group.

It seems worth while to underline the cunning (and sometimes downright perverted) aspect of certain cleverer psychopaths. These cunning psychopaths find a great pleasure in hurting, scandalising, and spreading discord. This pleasure will be even more intense if the object of attack is a source of respect to others. This is what makes The Samaritans a perfect target. If the psychopath cannot spread dissension among The Samaritans, he can try to discredit the organisation by slandering the work of the group, by the use of violence against one branch of the organisation, or by trying to push Samaritans to the use of force themselves. Having achieved this, he will claim that The Samaritans are not at all what they claim to be . . . He can try to make the group spend large sums of money (for example by making frequent reversed-charge calls), or to monopolise their time endlessly (by repeated telephone calls) – in short, to sabotage the organisation by every means at his disposal. These cases are extreme and fortunately rare, but can be a cause of real damage to the organisation. The best attitude to adopt to counter this behaviour and render it harmless seems to be one of strict neutrality. The least show of irritability on the part of Samaritans can feed the destructive force within these psychopaths. But equally dangerous would be lack of firmness or useless tolerance of their attacks. From this it is clear what a delicate matter it is to choose the right attitude. Those volunteers who are less experienced must first learn to refuse to deal with these problems and to refer them to those with more experience (Director, Samaritan-in-Charge).

The means at the disposal of The Samaritans

During their training, the new volunteers have an assortment of methods at their disposal. They can listen to potted case histories which expose problems already encountered with psychopaths. In this way they can get an idea of what it is all about, how these critical situations arise, and the consequences of the errors already committed. They can also learn how necessary it is to prepare oneself to avoid these situations. Above all, the various types of 'role-play' have an immense advantage by giving them an opportunity to play an active part. If during one of these role-plays the volunteer falls effectively into one of these traps, the question of why the trap worked should immediately be raised. Rarely (except in the case of a very skilful liar) is it the client's fault. Usually the volunteer will at this time have certain questions to ask himself:

What is his idea about his role as a Samaritan? Does he perhaps think that he must be able to do everything to help all the clients, and that the greater the effort the Samaritan's course of action demands, the better it must be?

Is it his sensitivity which led him to perceive too keenly the need of the client for more pity or interest, and caused him to lose his own capacity to evaluate the situation calmly?

Does he have a certain naïveté which renders him incapable of even conceiving of the existence of the means used by psychopaths arising out of their total lack of scruple and regard for others?

Does he panic in the face of blackmail?

Does he lack the training to reflect on the long-term consequences of the help given, and have too short-sighted a view of the interest of the client?

Is it a fact that he likes to feel needed? This is a very natural feeling for a person beginning Samaritan work, since something was required to give him the impulse to offer himself. If he can recognise the existence of this tendency in himself, without guilt, that can contribute one of the most essential stages in his development.

Does he suffer from an inability to say 'no' firmly but without aggressiveness? This can certainly be acquired only with experience and through total conviction.

Many other questions can be asked as the role-playing exercise becomes more and more developed and detailed. For the volunteer to learn to question himself in a positive manner – that is to say with the aim of understanding the problem better, without systematically accusing or torturing himself – can be a difficult task. A totally new and different way of thinking is sometimes necessary. To a new volunteer this exercise might seem unnecessarily painful, even frightening. Nevertheless, if he directs himself in this manner and if he is also helped by those who are experienced and of goodwill, he will quickly see the benefits that result from such instruction. He will soon see that his case is far from unique, and that many others – perhaps all – will have the same problems and that, by discussing them, they can often be effectively overcome.

For certain volunteers, their reluctance to question themselves in the preparation classes may come from an exaggerated fear of seeming inadequate in the eyes of others. But to refuse to face this questioning can only aggravate the fear, isolate the person from the group, and exaggerate the difficulties of the task. Thus the instruction of these anxious applicants requires that those who help them use great tact, take sufficient time before setting them to work, and encourage them more actively to develop a sense of self-confidence. If, on the other hand, others do not see the necessity to question themselves in this manner, this could be the result of a sense of false confidence. These applicants consider that they have already done enough self-questioning to meet successfully all the circumstances which might arise. Sometimes it is especially difficult and delicate to integrate these applicants into the team, and in this case it is more a question of slowing down their initiative without shaking their convictions too much. It is, perhaps, reasonable to allow them to face a real situation and make mistakes. After this, those who have made mistakes, and who are honest enough to admit it, can have a fruitful discussion with those Samaritans assigned to help them. These should not judge severely but, on the contrary, by being friendly and positive, should integrate them into the team without risk of further error. In certain cases, unfortunately, it seems from experience impossible to integrate new applicants successfully into the team, and their exclusion from The Samaritans should be decided.

Practice has shown (and we have also just seen) how important group discipline is within The Samaritans, particularly where psychopaths are concerned. Learning to work as a team instils a natural reflex of delegating responsibilities to the most competent, whenever this is judged necessary, or at least asking for advice without hesitation. Perhaps it is a training-ground for a certain modesty? It also teaches a respect for discipline: volunteers should under no circumstances undertake, without warning, any hasty action which contravenes the common mind of the group, even if they think themselves more capable of judging the problem than others. This is not to say, of course, that each member must obey blindly without having his personal opinion. When there is disagreement, discussion and debate should be encouraged. But this must precede any action, so that, when action is taken, it will be in a coherent manner, making it impossible for the psychopath to find occasion to sow discord amongst The Samaritans.

Of course, all volunteers may make mistakes with psychopaths, letting themselves be manipulated and abused. In such cases the Directors and the Samaritans-in-Charge have an essential function.

It would be highly regrettable for a volunteer who has realised his mistake, especially when dealing with a particularly tricky psychopath who has disillusioned him, if he became discouraged and lost confidence in the efficacy of Samaritan work. It would be equally regrettable if he became exaggeratedly suspicious in the hope of defending himself from a repetition of this experience. He should seek an interview with someone more experienced than himself, as this can sort things out and restore his confidence. But after many experiences, sometimes unhappy, isn't the development of a good sense of humour the best protection of the volunteer? Once he has gone beyond this stage of disillusionment, he realises that he cannot do everything, or succeed with every client, but that what he does is 'not so bad'.

Dangerous sentimentality – Chad Varah

How do so many psychopaths get accepted as clients in the first place, in spite of our precautions?

They have allies within the branch. Not usually fellow-psychopaths – few of these wangle their way in, and none remains long undetected – but muddleheaded sentimentalists who can be manipulated into breaking the rules. These are as dangerous as the psychopaths, and should be eliminated promptly.

Slavery degrades men to the extent of making them love it.

MARQUIS DE VAUVENARGUES

'Is there anybody out there?' – REX CANNON

This must be the agonizing cry of many despairing persons who find that life seems no longer to have any purpose: 'Who can understand, to whom can I turn, who has time for me? I am trapped in this dark endless tunnel of misery. Is there anyone anywhere?'

It has been realised for some time, as a result of a National Opinion Poll, that over 90% of the population know about The Samaritans but sadly, most are not fully aware of what we have to offer. Great strides have been made over recent years to create a more positive awareness of the support available, twenty-four hours day and night, in our 187 Branches.

The profile is being raised through a planned development in the media. Whilst the traditional forms of press coverage are vital to extend our message, the more personal style of Radio and TV interviews give the opportunity to impart the deeper feelings of Befriending. This was clearly illustrated by the immediate interest and response of the national TV and radio networks, when a 62-second commercial film was created for cinema audiences in Great Britain. Over 60% of filmgoers are under the age of 25 and the steady increase of suicide among young people in this age group has caused great concern.

This powerful film was produced with a background of music from 'The Wall' by Pink Floyd and earned the first 15 certificate to be given to a commercial advertising film. It also won the 1986 Design and Art Direction Silver award for the Best Public Service cinema commercial and a Gold award at the 1986 Cannes 'International du Film Publicitaire' Festival.

The impact of this deeply moving film 'Is there anybody out there?' produced immediate interest and response from the national network of TV and radio. The media coverage together with a cinema audience of over 2 million in 10 weeks has done much to encourage more lonely, frightened and desperate people to come to The Samaritans before taking that final step.

A new film 'Time to Talk' has recently been scripted, performed and filmed by the Children's Film Unit; a talented and highly skilled team of young people, who have already made a number of feature films, seen on the national TV network. This sensitive film was commissioned by The Samaritans, to be launched in 1987 as part of a complete educational pack to cover many aspects of young people's problems.

It may seem that concern is being mainly directed at the young – this is not so. Much thought and activity is being given to the needs of the elderly, prisons, hospitals and particularly those many people in the middle age groups who make up such a distressing number of those recorded as 'death by suicide'.

As one of many projects, a campaign is being launched to cover the London Underground and, for the first time, visitors to London and the many thousands of daily commuters will be constantly aware that there is 'Somebody out there' 24 hours a day.

New Dimensions – Barbara Espey and Sally Casper

Now that Lifeline, established in jails in the USA by Samaritans, is ten years old, it might perhaps be regarded as an *old* dimension, along with the Festival Branch in England, and Arnold the 'bus for Samaritan work in the open, but for the fact that it seems still to be confined to the USA, where our colleagues are very innovative without departing from our principles. The pioneer was the Revd. David Hogarth, Chaplain at the Charles Street jail in Boston, Mass., who has been Director of Lifeline in Boston since it began and has assisted each new Lifeline. The President of Samsusa, Barbara Espey, writes:

During 1986 The Samaritan volunteers met weekly with their colleagues, the Lifeline inmates who are the barred befrienders at the Charles Street jail in Boston, and at the jails in Lawrence, Salem and Barnstable. Each quarter, the

Samaritan members of all Lifeline programs join together and meet to offer each other encouragement, support and insight.

The inmate Lifeline members participate in the process of seeking out, identifying and befriending the suicidal, helpless, alienated and desperate among the thousands of new arrivals at the jails during the year.

Lifeline has played a signal role in the sheriffs' commitment to reducing the risk of suicide. The frequency of completed suicide has been reduced by 82 per cent since The Samaritans' work at the Charles Street jail began in 1978. There have been 6 completed suicides at Charles Street, rather than the 48 that the National Institute of Justice statistics indicate normally happen in a county institution of its size.

In 1983, Governor Dukakis appointed a Special Commission to Investigate Suicides in Municipal Lockups. This commission with active Samaritan participation has had public hearings and numerous meetings. As a result, legislation and public reports focusing on the reduction of suicide risks behind bars is anticipated.

Sally Casper writes: Samaritan volunteers meet weekly with Lifeline, a group of inmates selected and trained to befriend depressed and potentially suicidal men in the Lawrence Jail and House of Correction. The suicide rate behind bars is estimated to be 16 times higher than the rate in the general population. Lifeline is Sheriff Charles Reardon's official program for reducing the number of suicides in the Essex County jails.

Beyond the reach of The Samaritans' lifelines is the suicide attempt that occurs in a police lock-up – usually a young man picked up for drunk driving or another alcohol-related offense. Through the Massachusetts Criminal Justice Training Academy, The Samaritans offer an all-day training course several times a year for police, correction officers and youth service workers, on how to identify suicide risk and respond in a lifesaving way.

Safe Place – Sally Casper and Carolyn Benedict Drew

Another new dimension pioneered in USA is Safe Place. This is the name given to groups which meet regularly to provide support for those who have lost a friend or family member through suicide.

Groups are currently meeting under the sponsorship of the following branches: The Samaritans of Rhode Island, The Samaritans of Merrimack Valley, and The Samaritans of Albany. At Andover in Merrimack Valley, 51 men and women who had lost a family member through suicide made use of Safe Place in the first 18 months since it started in July 1982.

Carolyn Benedict Drew, Director of The Samaritans of Providence, RI, USA adds:

Safe Place meets one evening per month. However, we are considering meeting twice a month. We do not ask participants to contract a time with us nor do we insist that members speak at a meeting. We open our meeting with a statement and we give each member a copy of *After Suicide* by John Hewitt for their keeping. Because we strongly believe in confidentiality, we do not directly contact survivors. The State Medical Examiner sends a copy of *Grief After Suicide*, and informs family members of Safe Place. We send out monthly reminders to all people who have ever attended a Safe Place meeting, and we advertise Safe Place in all media community calendars.

The facilitators of Safe Place are totally non-directive and are there to open and close the meeting, to share in the survivor's pain and to give members permission to have the feelings that follow a suicide of a loved one. Personally, I strongly believe that death by suicide bereavement groups need to be separate from all other groups sharing bereavement because suicide remains socially unacceptable and the group members need to share, not only their feelings, but perhaps their visual memories of finding a family member who has hanged him or herself or shot him or herself. Death by suicide is the cruellest death of all and therefore members must be allowed to show their anger, share their forever 'whys', and discuss their guilt in a safe place.

Facilitating Safe Place is one of the most difficult parts of my job. Therefore I believe it is paramount that the facilitator has a network of support following every meeting.

It is my hope that someone, somewhere will have the time

to organise a national meeting for facilitators of bereavement groups.

Lifeline Triumph – David Hogarth

In January 1985 I learnt that all the recommendations of the Governor's Commission on Cell-block Suicide had been legislated the last day of the 1984 General Court; the first legislation in the world on cell-block suicide.

Our three recommendations were accepted:

1) Every local police officer in Massachusetts has to be trained in suicide assessment and intervention.
2) All local lockups must be fitted with plastic over bars, have no horizontal pipes or projections, and have audio monitors which have to be heard rather than TV monitors which aren't watched.
3) There must be a permanent recording of any suicide gesture, threat or attempt by an arrestee.

I spent a frenzied time training 50 people to do the training.

If a person attempts or commits suicide in an unmodified cell after 1986, the jurisdiction is liable for negligence.

Within three hours of an inmate's arrival, the jail scans the suicide file (7000 cases a year) enabling us to take precautions.

Ancient Menander accounted him happy that had but met the shadow of a true friend.

MONTAIGNE

A Letter to doctors – J. L. T. BIRLEY

Dear Doctor,

If you were feeling depressed or irritable or bewildered by unusual and perhaps shameful feelings; or if work was beginning to pile up; or your evening drink was becoming longer and earlier; how easy would it be for you to sit in your surgery and go in to talk to your busy bustling, competent-looking self, with twenty more patients still in the waiting-room?

Many people find it very daunting. They may feel the doctor's bustle is partly real, partly protective. If they did start to talk, or worse still, to cry, would the doctor be prepared to listen? He might be embarrassed or feel out of his depth and bring the interview to an end with a reassuring or dismissive comment and perhaps a prescription for tranquillisers. Faced with these possibilities, many depressed people keep silent or look elsewhere. But the most desperate do go to their doctors. Barraclough found that two-thirds of those who committed suicide visited their GP during the previous month and 40 per cent during the week prior to their death.

The Samaritans are not doctors – although a number of doctors are also Samaritans. They do not bustle, they listen, usually invisibly and anonymously on the telephone. They have plenty of time. They are trained to talk about and accept their callers' feelings of hopelessness and self-destruction. They do not diagnose. They have no power to go against their callers' own wishes. Paradoxically, it is their powerlessness which gives them their strength.

Samaritans need to be seen as confidential and separate from the medical profession. But they are eager to co-operate with them and are fully aware of the risks of undermining their callers' relationships with their own doctors. A common 'assignment' is persuading a caller to consult or return to the doctor. Sometimes a Samaritan will offer to act as intermediary – a delicate task as a doctor may be offended by the implication that his patient has found it easier to talk to a Samaritan than to himself.

But referral need not and should not be all in one direction. Many doctors refer their patients to The Samaritans, or suggest that they get in touch with them.

These are just some of the ways in which The Samaritans and the medical profession can work together. And, Doctor; if you *are* feeling depressed, irritable or in any way as I described at the beginning of this letter, you are welcome to call The Samaritans yourself. Many doctors, including psychiatrists, do so. For all sorts of reasons, doctors often find it difficult to get this sort of help from each other.

Yours sincerely, JIM BIRLEY

A principal fruit of friendship is the ease and discharge of the fulness and swellings of the heart, which passions of all kinds cause and induce.

FRANCIS BACON

They speak for themselves – EMILY MEIR
2nd series

No fixed abode

I can't go on like this, you know. It's just not possible, I feel as if, somewhere, there's another me, and I think he must love me, but I can't find him. I walk and I walk and I think I'm getting somewhere and I'm not. I can't rest, I can't get into a train or a bus. People stare at me so angrily and I can't rest anywhere.

It's only 10.30 so I've got eleven and a half hours' walking to do today. Feel my head! Feel the top of my head! It's burning, burning. What am I going to do?

I need some sleep, but I can't settle down anywhere . . . I'd like soup, please, coffee makes my head burn. I don't want any doctors. I just want to sort out who I am. These last two or three days I haven't been myself at all. But who is myself? I don't want any medicine – I just want to get clear in my mind . . . I've been in hospital. I've been in that one down the road and I'm no different, am I? I still don't know who I am! I'll just sit here and have my drink and not be a bother to anyone.

Pregnancy

I think I'm pregnant. How can I find out for sure? Shall I have to give my name if I go to the clinic? I'm only 15. I'm still at school. Will my mother and father get to know? He'll kill me. I look older than I am because I'm tall. I went to this party, see, and I'm not used to having so much to drink . . . It was my first time for sex. I never intended to do it . . . I wouldn't use the pill. You look so cheap if you do, as though you were expecting to have sex any time. Where is this clinic? Could someone go with me? I daren't tell my mother – she'd die. What shall I say to them? . . . I want to stay on at school for my

'A' levels. I want to be a Social Worker. Funny, isn't it? Ironical?

They've all got knives

It's my boy I'm ringing about. He's thirteen, but he looks a lot older. He's tall and very attractive to the girls unfortunately, so he's having a terrible time at his Comprehensive School.

One day last week, one of the girls came after him and groped him. He hates that, but I've taught him never to start a fight and never to strike girls, so he just walked away. Well, her friend took that as an insult and went up and hit him. She said the whole gang of boys would be after him. They were – they lay in wait for him after school and he had to run all the way home . . . I wasn't back from work, so he couldn't get in and had to go to a neighbour. The trouble is, you see, they all have knives these days and they're quick to use them . . . He was terrified of going in this morning . . .

If I tell the head teacher they will have it in for him even more and the police have enough on their hands already in this area. I tell you, it's more like a battlefield than a school these days!

Like a leper

I must see a priest – I'm desperate. Have you got a priest there? I can't talk to anyone at work – I have too important a position and too many people working for me . . . At home I've been terrible to my friend too. You see I'm convinced I've got AIDS . . . I've always had a phobia about dying since my Mother died while I was abroad on holiday. She died of cancer and I ought to have been with her . . . Now I'm afraid of dying in isolation – not even having my friends round me.

The friend I live with pooh-poohs my anxiety. He says it's not the least likely, but he's not gay. I don't sleep with him, so I sleep with other men from time to time. I've been to a Special Clinic for the symptoms I've got and the Doctor said I had some infection. He gave me antibiotics and told me to come back when I'd finished the course. He didn't even tell me not to have sex. Would he have told me if I had AIDS? Could they be careless and miss it? Oh, What can I do? What can I do? . . .

With this horrible AIDS I'm sure I'm going to die and be

wrapped in a plastic sheet . . . It's just like being a leper! I must see a priest. Can you find me one?

Are peacocks unlucky?

Do you think peacocks are unlucky? The thing is you see, I'm thinking of buying my daughter a vase with a peacock on it, but I've heard peacocks bring bad luck. You see my father lives in India, and he has a big supermarket with all sorts of jewellery and pottery and so on, and the business isn't doing too well. He thinks it's because of the peacock vases he has. Just the eye on it. The eye seems to watch you and follow you about. Some say it's an evil influence – what would you feel about it?

Then I thought of getting my nieces Chinese vases instead, with similar patterns, but then I thought maybe they'd like the same pattern as each other. I can't make up my mind . . . I suppose I am a bit depressed and homesick! Could I really come in and talk to someone?

Living together

It's difficult to know where to start now I've got here. How much notice should one take of public opinion? Does it matter what the neighbours think? I suppose it's the legal consequences that scare me really.

Well I'm in my 40s (not really) and my sister and I live in the family home . . . I'm quite a successful business man and she used to be a fashion model. I was divorced several years ago and my sister is single. Since my divorce we've lived together and I do mean lived together. We're very happy. I think she feels safe with me, because she had some traumatic experiences earlier on. She doesn't worry about our situation at all, but I do.

She's in her thirties; suppose later on she regrets not being married and having children? Or suppose someone notices one day when we're off guard?

Today the window cleaners came and I thought, suppose they notice there's only one double bed and her nightdress is on one side of it and my pyjamas on the other?

She says I'm silly. I could have had a girlfriend sleeping with me – but I don't know. It's the little things that betray you.

When we went on holiday I suddenly realised our passports said Mr and Miss 'Brown' . . . I just laughed and told the porter they'd made a silly mistake, but he couldn't have cared less.

I came to you here of course because it's a long way from home.

Like a monkey

It's taken an enormous effort for me to get here and now I don't know where to begin. Well, it goes a very long way back to when I was thirteen and still at home in Malaysia. I was at school and the teacher asked me to read aloud in class. I was ever so nervous and it made me want to giggle . . . The teacher shouted at me. She said 'You look like a monkey' . . . I felt so terrible I ran home and never told anyone, but I couldn't forget it. I got through school somehow and I came to England to study accountancy, but I can't concentrate on my exams at all because I feel so ugly and horrible. I took a course in Elocution before I left home. I've been to a psychiatrist. I've attended a Social Skills Group. I've had hypnotherapy. I've even been to a clairvoyant, but none of it makes any difference . . . I've tried to hang myself, but it was so painful I couldn't do it. I don't know how to go on living!

My parents couldn't help. They are just simple peasants. It's all they could do to bring up their eight children materially. They wouldn't understand what it was about at all . . . I have no one. No one.

Being a mother in 1986

It's about my boy. He's a very good boy. He goes to church. He teaches in the Methodist Sunday School, where they've got a strong Youth movement. He's not violent and I don't think he takes drugs but he has got some very dubious friends. One of them was expelled from school. And they have such wild parties! You can't imagine what parties are like nowadays . . .

His father and I are divorced and his father has remarried. Well, his father let him use his flat for a party while he was away on holiday. I went because I dreaded what I might see – It was a riot. People gate-crashing. People bringing huge bottles of rum and vodka . . . Girls. Fights. Noise – unbelievable! In the end I had to call the police to control them . . . And he's only 16!

Now he's just gone on holiday with a party of boys to Greece. They've taken a villa. No, there's no adult with them. We parted badly because he's so angry with me for making a fuss about it. I do try to be a tolerant modern mother, honestly I do, but there's so much danger about now . . . When he'd gone I looked round his room and I found hundreds and hundreds of cigarette ends. Now isn't that funny, because I've never even seen him smoke!

I'm on my own now and I've enough worries without all this. I don't even get the money for his school uniform till after I've bought it . . . Still, while he's away, I can live on much less – I've lived from Monday to Friday on one pound – I couldn't have done that if he were here, could I?

All for love

My name is Jehan and I come from India. My father is very rich . . . I was to be a student of Politics and Economics, but I met this girl in a shoe shop and fell in love with her. She's a very attractive girl. We went out several times and then I asked her to live with me. I found out that she had been a prostitute, but she told me she'd had a wretched life and been in care since childhood, so I felt very sorry for her and I thought it would all change once we were married.

She said she had only done it to escape. Still my father was very angry and he will have nothing more to do with me. But I love Rachel – yes – she is English – I absolutely adore her. So I took various jobs – I worked as a waiter and we managed for a while. Then one day she disappeared from the Northern town where we were living. I searched our old haunts and I found her living with a friend of mine. He didn't know she had been with me. 'Oh, she's just a bit on the side,' he said. So I took her back, and I begged my mother to help me financially. She gave me a thousand pounds. I thought then Rachel would be happy and satisfied, but she's gone again and I can't find her. See my feet are bleeding with walking the streets looking for her. And I found out only yesterday from another girl that she's on drugs – the heavy stuff. But I've got to find her. I must help her. When my grandmother dies I could give her all the money she could wish for. I'm a bit weak because I've had nothing to eat since she went, but that doesn't matter. I just want to find her. Here's her photograph. Isn't she lovely?

Looking on the bright side

I came to tell you how I went on at Guy's. You kindly sent me there in a taxi when I had pains on Saturday. Well, the doctor said I have adhesions from my old operations. He gave me an injection and told me to come back in three days if it isn't better and be opened up. So they'd have to unpack all my insides again.

They said maybe I don't eat enough of the right food. Well, I eat what I can afford, don't I? And that's not much on an invalidity pension!

I've got my own little council flat now and I'm really proud of it, but you do need a bit of humanity . . . At least when you live in a hostel you meet other people at mealtimes. Do you know, when I first went there I actually stood outside my kitchen door the first morning waiting for breakfast to arrive. I know it was daft, but I'd done it for so many years.

No, what I really hate is hanging about there all day with nothing to do. So I've joined an agency for part-time work and that will give me something to get up for every morning – just going up there to see if there's any work. I'll get up at 5.30 and wash and shave and dress and go and see what there is! Even if there's nothing I'll have something to get up for!

Mother says I'm too young

I'm eighteen. I've got a little girl of three. I'm not married. Now I'm pregnant again. I wanted to get married the first time. Now I want to even more but my mother won't let me. She says I'm too young . . . It's the same boy friend I've had all the time; he's the father of both children . . . He's very good because I was only fifteen the first time and he could have washed his hands of me, but he was prepared to take the responsibility then and he's prepared to marry me now . . . He wants to marry me.

He lives in the same block of flats but not in the same flat. I share a flat with a girlfriend. He's got a good job and he can afford to keep me.

We want to be married but my mother says I must see more of the world first . . . I don't think I'll see much of the world with two young children anyway – whether I'm married or not. I'm going to see my doctor this afternoon – he's 90% certain I'm pregnant . . . Why can't my mother let me lead my life my way?

The morning after

I've got the shakes. I don't know where I'm supposed to be. I got arrested for drunk and disorderly on Friday and I spent the night in the police station. I was supposed to be somewhere at 10.30 this morning . . . The police gave me an address to go to for drying out. They made an appointment for me. Now I've forgotten where it is . . . If I don't get some treatment soon I know I'll kill myself with the drink and I'm only thirty-two.

I haven't been on Social Security. Up to eight months ago I was in the Royal Navy, but I've gone to pieces since my mother and father died. I'm from Scotland – I don't know London at all.

I'll never find my way about. When I woke up I was sitting on a park bench and I didn't know whether it was morning or evening . . . I had to ask. I felt such a fool.

Oh, look, here's the bit of paper the police gave me in my pocket. It's some unit for alcoholics. I've got a bit of money but I'll never find the way. Will you ring them please and tell them why I'm late? And can I have a wash first?

Let down

It's always happening to me, but I feel just terrible every time. I'm twenty-three and I met a boy at the weekend, very good-looking and attractive. He asked me out and was very pleasant. He seemed to like me a lot, too. He made a date for the weekend. He even suggested we should go on holiday together. He told me to ring him nearer the weekend.

When I did ring him he was quite different. He was so cold and distant – a different boy altogether – so detached. He said he felt tired and wouldn't be able to make it. He was so tired and so busy. It could be true, but he was as cold as if we'd never met. Do you think it's because I didn't have sex with him that first time? I said not on the first date – sometime later maybe.

Do you think it was that? It's true I'd got to be the one who rang him. He didn't ring me.

I feel so hurt and upset. It had all sounded so lovely. This sort of thing is always happening to me . . . boys letting me down like this. You wonder whether it's worth struggling on at all . . . Is it me? What is it about me?

Rescue?

We've come down from Manchester on the night coach. We had to wait four hours for one, but the children are very good. They'd already had their baths . . . We were in the bathroom when my husband started shouting. He began to knock me about again and started hitting them. Well, he's had me in hospital before, and I wasn't going to let them suffer too. I just said 'we're going' – and we left.

We've been in a Women's Aid hostel before, but he found us so that's why we've come down to London. The children's name isn't the same as mine.

He's my second husband, you see. Tom, my elder child, was born when I was still single, and the little girl is the child of my first marriage. I'm twenty-four . . . The children are really quite grown up for their age – they know we're going to a hostel. They've had a bit of sleep in the coach. Could you get us into a hostel, please?

Fear of violence

I look a civilised man, don't I? You would never believe the things I do – I'm afraid I've ruined my relationship this time. When I'm drunk I get very wild and say bitter things . . . I'm homosexual and I'm very jealous – once I'm drunk I'm beyond all control . . . This time I threw a TV at my boyfriend and knocked him down. I'm scared I'll kill him in one of my rages.

It's got to the stage where he's terrified of me. He's so depressed lately he's been tearing out his hair in handfuls . . . Now he's left me again and I don't think he'll come back this time. But he hasn't taken his things . . . I don't know where he is. No, he hasn't a job. He lost that through me. I kept 'phoning him at work where he was night porter and I followed him to work. Naturally they got fed up and sacked him.

I know how badly I need treatment but I'm afraid if I go away from here I'll never have the courage to come back. I know my jealousy is insane – How can I stop it?

There is no man that imparteth his griefs to his friend but he grieveth the less.

FRANCIS BACON

How to start a Branch – VANDA SCOTT

Before being recognised as a BI* Branch, there are 5 stages in development. This enables BI to maintain the required high standard of care for the suicidal and despairing. BI must formally approve each change of stage and this is usually achieved through visits made by the Area Rep.** It is hoped that the Area Rep's visits will be sponsored by the developing branch.*** However, BI is wholly aware that this may not always be possible. Applications for help in this matter can be made to the Chairman. At each stage BI will supply as much support and detailed information as is possible, in order to enable a developing branch to move forward. The whole process is co-ordinated by the Chairman through the Area Rep.

Stages of development

1. Initial contact by interested person.
2. Exploratory Group
3. Foundation Group
4. Probationary Branch
5. A Branch

Stages of Development Explained

1. *Contact by person(s) wishing information on how to start a Branch*

   All initial contact is referred to the Chairman who will:

   (a) send an introductory letter detailing the organisation's

* Befrienders International Samaritans Worldwide

** For 'Area Rep' read 'Area Representative or person approved by B.I. Chairman'

*** For Branch, also read Centre

aims together with a history of BI, a brochure and general information.

(b) put the person in touch with the Area Rep.

If it is appropriate the Area Rep will ask this person to form an Exploratory Group. This stage may be eliminated if the interested person is known to BI. In this case the Chairman will start the process at Stage 2 and ask the person to form an Exploratory Group.

2. *Exploratory Group*

This group is comprised of at least 6 people from the community, all of whom will have an interest in starting a Samaritan Branch in their area. It will be given access to further documented information and the Samaritan film. It will assess the real need for such a branch by talking to local people already in touch with distressed people e.g. charity organisations, social workers, priests, etc., and, wherever possible, search out statistics on suicide and attempted suicide.

If a need is confirmed then this group, before proceeding further, must agree to:

(a) abide by the 7 Principles and 7 Practices of the Samaritans.

(b) abide by the Constitution.

The Area Rep will give a detailed, full explanation of (a) and (b) to the group.

The group is now ready to take the next two steps:

(a) assess the capability of recruiting 15 suitable volunteers prepared to put time, energy and commitment into initially starting a new Branch. (The assessment may include the Exploratory Group. It is important that the group realise that all Samaritans must have attended a preparation course. It is also important to realise that not all organisers necessarily make good Samaritans – but both are equally needed when it comes to founding a Branch. A degree of self-honesty is needed when making this assessment!).

(b) assess the capability of recruiting enough volunteers from the area to eventually run a branch operating 24 hours a day and with at least 70 volunteers.

If the interest of the group is still high and the previous criteria have been met, at the discretion of the Area Rep the group will be asked to form a Foundation Group.

3. *A Foundation Group*
   A foundation Group is comprised of at least 6 people who, having studied the findings of the Exploratory Group, agree there is a need for a Samaritan Branch in the area. This group will agree to abide by the 7 Principles and 7 Practices and accept the BI Constitution.

   The function of the Foundation Group
   The function of this group is to agree to:
   (a) locate premises;
   (b) design and obtain equipment and furnishings for the centre;
   (c) decide on the type of advertising needed to attract callers and to advertise a PR evening and opening of the centre;
   (d) programme each item needed to be covered before opening the Probationary Branch;
   (e) budget projection;
   (f) raise funds;
   (g) initiate a public relations evening to heighten community interest and attract potential Samaritan volunteers;
   (h) run a Preparation Course;
   (i) liaise with the Area Rep.

   In order to achieve the above it is usual for the group to elect, from amongst itself, a member who will act as a Co-ordinator.

   A Co-ordinator is the person who will liaise with the group, organise meetings and liaise with the Area Rep. It is not necessarily the person who will eventually become Director of the Probationary Branch. The Co-ordinator needs primarily to be someone with initiating, management and organising skills. The Co-ordinator will be responsible for carrying out, or delegating, all work associated with the opening of a Probationary Branch and for seeking a person suitable to be Director.

By now it will be realised that many areas have to be covered in order to initiate and open a Probationary Branch. Whilst many areas being covered overlap, for reason of clarity, it is thought best for a Foundation Group to address the needs in two phases. *Phase I* would cover the practical needs of planning and opening a Probationary Branch. *Phase II* would cover the recruitment of volunteers – the running of the Preparation Course and eventual service to be given to callers.

Phase I

(a) *Location of premises*
The Probationary Branch must have a centre from which to work. This will either be within a large building or in premises standing alone. Ideally it will be:
 (i) centrally located within the anticipated catchment area for callers;
 (ii) located so as to give the caller as much anonymity as possible. (Callers are often shy about standing outside a branch and ringing the bell or they may fear being seen by someone they know.) It is suggested that consideration be given to premises in a side street, off a main road, or in a building much frequented by people going about their ordinary business;
 (iii) located in a position likely to attract the maximum number of callers. From experience this is unlikely to be a building associated with sectarian or religious groups;
 (iv) located where both callers and volunteers will feel physically safe;
 (v) near a car park if the branch is in a country which relies heavily on the car as transport;
 (vi) near public transport terminals, or in a location easily accessible by public transport, if the branch is in a country relying heavily on public transport.

(b) *The design of the centre*
Every Samaritan Branch obviously has different needs when taking into account the fact that BI serves so many

people in so many countries throughout the world. The design of a centre will alter, e.g. if the service is heavily weighted towards callers being able to 'drop in'. In that case more interview facilities will be needed and a smaller operations rooms would suffice.

Below is a specimen of what is considered necessary in an ideal situation for a branch operating both a telephone and interview service.

(i) Telephone operations room
(ii) Interview rooms for face-to-face befriending
(iii) Reception/waiting area
(iv) Volunteers' relaxing area and facilities (kitchen, toilet and shower)
(v) Administration area
(vi) Training room (optional extra)

A centre should have sufficient space to be partitioned into separate rooms. The following are suggestions for the layout:

(i) *Telephone operations room* This is a closed-access area to all but Samaritans and therefore can be situated away from the main entrance/reception area in a location where privacy and quietness can be maintained.

This room contains the emergency telephones (preferably located in sound-proof booths), an administration telephone (for contacting the leader-on-duty, director, ambulance, consultants, etc), the callers' records (available therefore to the Samaritan on duty but with the utmost security). Space should be available for folding beds (overnight duty requirement) to be erected and an extra chair or two for extra volunteers in the operations room who are not on telephone duty but working.

Requirements: 2 emergency telephones
2 telephone sound-proof booths
2 desks
2 chairs
1 administrative telephone
a table and extra chairs
filing cabinets for callers' records

2 folding beds
notice boards
bookshelf
card index boxes

(ii) *Interview rooms* Situated close to the main entrance hall to allow callers as much anonymity as is possible on their arrival at the centre.

2 easy chairs
coffee table
plants and pictures

(iii) *Reception/waiting area* Near the entrance of the centre to be as friendly, homely and as private as possible.

(iv) *Volunteers' relaxing area* This should be situated away from the public area and have facilities for volunteers to shower, relax and make coffee in private.

(v) *Administration Area* for director, secretary, treasurer and other volunteers with administrative responsibilities to continue without disturbing the main function of the centre. This area requires storage space for stationery, publicity material, plus:

desks and chairs
typewriter
filing cabinets
shelves
notice boards

(vi) *Meeting room* (optional extra) If space is available a training/meeting room is great to have, to hold approximately 25 people. Chairs and folding tables are necessary, plus a blackboard.

If only one undivided area is available and all aspects of Samaritan work have to take place in this area, then the emergency telephone should be positioned as far away as possible from the administrative area and callers being befriended in person. Visual divisions such as curtains, notice boards and filing cabinets should be used to isolate the telephone emergency area from the rest of the work in the Centre.

(c) *The type and frequency of advertising for callers*
It is good to have someone with advertising experience in your area as a member of the Foundation Group. From experience posters are the most reasonable in cost as a form of advertising but fliers in newspapers, brochures in offices and doctors' surgeries, advertisements in newspapers, television and radio interviews and advertising, are some of the other ways to get known in the community. The word 'suicide' should be included in all advertising.
Things to remember
(i) Always be sure your advertisements are absolutely honest. Nothing is worse than for a caller who has read that the Samaritan Branch opening hours are 9 a.m.–10 p.m. and who plucks up all his or her courage to ring during those hours to find that there is no one there.
(ii) It is also important to be absolutely sure of the Probationary Branch's opening day before advertising the service. Painters can be delayed!
(iii) For Probationary Branches relying on the telephone, or even partially on the telephone, for callers' contact it is good to try and get an easily remembered telephone number e.g. 222333.

The Chairman's office has sample posters from some of our many branches throughout the world. If you are interested in seeing these then ask your Area Rep for further information.

It is believed that the service cannot work unless it is extensively advertised. Ideally the advertising would be as good as Coca Cola's but the frequency of advertising is usually dependent upon finance. It is desirable that this subject is addressed early on the agenda since without it there will probably be few callers and possibly few volunteers.

(d) *A programme*
From the outset it is advisable to have a programme detailing who is doing what job and when results can be expected, e.g. 'Mary enquiring about free advertising

local paper 5 May' and under 11 May 'Mary telling us whether free advertising possible.' So many events overlap leading to the first day of operation for the Probationary Branch and many things are going on simultaneously. Just as a Foundation Group needs a Co-ordinator so it needs a programme to co-ordinate dates for each item needing to be covered.

(e) *Budget projection*
The Foundation Group needs someone who is good with figures, a person who can project the amount of money needed for the overall cost of starting a Probationary Branch and running it for one year. The budget should include such items as the cost of advertising for callers and volunteers, the cost of the running a Preparation Course, the cost of rental of premises, the cost of public utilities, etc. Once the group knows the expected expenditure then it can address the question of how it will be raised.

(f) *Fund raising*
There are obviously many ways to raise funds stretching from holding jumble sales and raffles to someone giving the whole amount needed for the Probationary Branch to get started. The main thing to remember is that a Samaritan Branch is non-sectarian and non-religious, etc., and that any funds with 'strings attached' (that is funds given with provisos) must be considered very seriously before it is decided that they should be accepted.

People *do* like to know their donations or fund raising efforts are well used. It may be that donations can be raised with specific areas in mind, e.g. someone donates a desk or a filing cabinet or offers to pay the phone bill for one year; another, the rent, etc. Round Tables and Rotary Clubs have been generous to many of their respective local Samaritan Branches around the world.

Phase II

The recruitment of volunteers
There are several ways to recruit volunteers but experience has

proved that the best way seems to be to hold an Open Evening which is well-advertised to attract members of the public in the Area. At the Open Evening the Samaritan film is shown and a person, not necessarily the Co-ordinator, chairs the meeting and answers questions. At the end of the meeting it is advisable to have application forms for people to pick up and take home with them. When the form has been returned the interested person should be contacted *as soon as possible* (nothing puts a potential volunteer off more than not hearing from us for weeks!). At this point of contact an appointment is made for the person to meet and be interviewed by 2 of the Foundation Group.

What sort of person is a Samaritan volunteer?

'The Samaritan volunteer is accepted into the organisation not because he knows how to cope with someone who has taken an overdose, nor because of his experience in getting people down off roofs and window ledges from which they threaten to jump. He (or she) is not chosen for any particular abilities (useful though they may be and some volunteers have them), but for those human qualities that make a good friend, a good neighbour, a good person to have with you when you are in trouble. It is not so much what he does, but in BEING his own patient, tolerant, interested self that the Samaritan helps the caller most. Someone can usually be found to do things that require a particular knowledge or abilities, and the Samaritan is prepared to go to endless trouble about this, but he knows that his talent is friendship, and his unfailing concern is what he was engaged for and that this is the thing the majority of the clients need most.' (*The Samaritans in the 70's* by Chad Varah).

So the person who makes a 'good' volunteer, by definition of what Chad Varah has just said, is someone who is accepting and not judgmental; a listener rather than a doer; a person able to commit time and be on time, rather than a dreamer; a person able to hear a person and think 'given different circumstances in my life – that could be me.' A Samaritan is someone who can identify with a caller in a human way without being in any way condescending.

NB. When recruiting first-time volunteers for a new Probationary Branch it is tempting to accept all those volunteers who come forward. It is tempting, but volunteers must be turned away, as gently as is humanly possible, if they are thought to be in any way unsuitable.

When a Foundation Group has 15 volunteers then it is ready to commence a Preparation Course.

The Preparation Course

Once the Preparation Course is completed (or at the final session) arrangements are made for a second interview with 2 members of the Foundation Group for the potential volunteer. During the Preparation Course the volunteers will have had time to assess their own suitability and Foundation Group members will similarly have had the opportunity to assess the volunteer. This second interview is meant to assess whether the volunteer will continue and be a volunteer with the Probationary Branch and it is an opportunity for the Foundation Group to receive feedback with reference to the selection procedure and Preparation course. After the second interview and when the criteria of 15 volunteers has been met, a General Meeting is called by the Co-ordinator of the Foundation Group and all the new volunteers.

The General Meeting to select a Director for the Probationary Branch

The Co-ordinator chairs the general meeting which is held for the purpose of selecting a Director for the Probationary Branch. The Director will be expected to hold office for one year at a time but may be re-elected for further terms of office. It is usual that this period will not exceed 3 years but some branches use 5 years and others even longer.

Outline of the Director's role

The Director may, and is advised to, delegate various tasks, but he/she is ultimately responsible for:

(i) Being the Branch's public spokesman. The Director will inevitably lose his/her anonymity.

(ii) Adequate selection and training of volunteers.

(iii) Rostering of Samaritans and correct manning of phones.
(iv) Provision for on-going training.
(v) Selection of a deputy Director (not to be delegated).
(vi) Selection of competent Leaders (not to be delegated).
(vii) Leader training.
(viii) Arranging and chairing Leaders' Meeting.
(ix) Arranging and chairing Management Committee meetings.
(x) Presenting an Annual Report and the Annual General Meeting.
(xi) Ensuring that adequate financial records are kept.
(xii) Replying to correspondence.
(xiii) Seeking to advertise the Samaritan Service.
(xiv) Attending to the welfare of the Samaritan volunteers.
(xv) Providing regular reports on Branch progress to the B.I. Area Rep.
(xvi) Keeping the Area Rep informed of names of current volunteers.
(xvii) Raising funds.

The Director should:
(a) Be a committed person with time to attend to the running of the Centre;
(b) Have the ability to deal with volunteers;
(c) Have some administrative skills;
(d) Be able to compile letters and address an audience;
(e) Be able to operate in a professional manner.

The Director, once elected, is then ready to select his or her team of people who are called Leaders.

At this time it is wise to stress that a volunteer's first responsibility is to be a Samaritan volunteer who does a duty (at least 3½ hours) once a week. This duty involves complete availability to either see a caller face to face, or speak to a caller on the telephone. Any further work undertaken by a volunteer within the Branch will be extra to that duty. If the volunteer becomes overburdened then the 'further work' is given up in order to allow the Samaritan to concentrate on doing his or her weekly duty to the caller. *Nothing is regarded as more important than that of being a volunteer in contact with the caller.*

With this in mind the Director invites between 5 and 7 members of the volunteer group to become Leaders. It has been found that the Leadership system works better than any other when operating a Branch. Our work, of necessity, can become stressful. Often when a Samaritan has been closely in touch with a deeply distressed caller someone outside the situation is needed to assist in sorting through what the Samaritan has heard.

A Samaritan is not allowed to make decisions alone – it is too much of a responsibility to do so when our work deals with life and death. Samaritans are members of a team and for this reason it is advised that a Leader has another Leader to refer to when they, themselves, are on their weekly Samaritan Duty.

Leaders will be asked:

(a) Either to be in the centre, or be completely available at another telephone number, during a period of 12–24 hours per week.

(b) To get to know the volunteers on a Samaritans level, i.e. knowing the volunteers' strengths and weaknesses and getting the confidence of the volunteers so they may share any difficulties occurring in their personal lives.

(c) To assist in the co-ordination of the Branch by freely communicating with other Leaders any information that is important to the general well-being of the caller.

(d) To make sure that volunteers are aware of 'standing orders' regarding callers.

(e) To pass any information important to the caller from one volunteer on duty to the next and to check that information is passed and messages given between volunteers.

(f) To ring the Centre *once* during on-duty period or more frequently depending on what is happening at the Centre, or to be in the Centre and available for immediate consultation.

(g) To encourage Samaritans to discuss their duty period by asking about callers even though there may not have been a problem (never to accept that 'nothing has happened' without a query).

(h) Always to question the volunteer as to what the caller wanted and how the caller was feeling at the end of the call.
(i) To be ready to ask whether the necessary paper work concerning a caller has been done.
(j) To check the Log Book to make sure all the entries make sense, and all the entries are correct.
(k) To check messages or papers relating to all callers, especially those at risk.
(l) To make sure that callers who appear on the emergency notice are only there during their crisis period.
(m) To work closely with the filing clerks and to assist them in the correction of any filing mistakes, either by leaving a message for the volunteer or by ringing the volunteer.
(n) To attend Leaders' meetings.
(o) To convey any relevant comments or requests from such a meeting.
(p) To share such administrative duties as are necessary with the Director and other Leaders.
(q) To make personal contact with new probationary volunteers as soon as they are in the Centre; to make provision for their on-going training; to monitor their progress during their probationary period and to make sure they are fully assimilated into the system.

In summary, a Leader is responsible for all decisions, paper work, volunteers who are on duty, during the period he/she is on duty as a Leader. No other work within the Branch at the time should be undertaken by the Leader if it is detrimental to the work of *being* a Leader. It is the prime responsibility of the Leaders to ask questions, e.g. How did you help the caller? Do you think the caller will phone back? How are you feeling about the call?

Conclusion

The Foundation Group has now prepared the ground for opening a Probationary Branch. It has volunteers prepared; it has a centre; it has a Director and Leaders and publicity will be well under way advertising the forthcoming service and the opening date. The remaining task is to set up the office and to prepare the volunteers in office procedure. There is a lot of work involved and the following Aims of Branches summarises concisely the on-going commitment of a new Branch.

N.B. At each stage in the Foundation Group's development the group will be in touch via the Co-ordinator with the Area Rep and the service will not be allowed to advertise the opening day until the Area Rep is totally satisfied that the Foundation Group will be ready to 'go' and has approved the proposed Director.

Aims of Branches

All Branches should offer the following in their service for callers:

(1) Good advertisements with easy access by telephone, visit or letter.
(2) Anonymity for callers and volunteers (first names or a chosen first name used), and a serial number in place of a surname.
(3) Complete confidentiality.
(4) A non-religious, non-political stance.
(5) Referrals to other agencies or professionals for medical, practical or professional help if appropriate.
(6) Willingness to call a suicidal person at the request of a reliable third party if the risk seems high and the person agrees.
(7) Primary concern for those in danger of suicide but also befriending the lonely, depressed, isolated and those who cannot cope at the time of contact.
(8) No charge for help.
(9) Adherence to the Seven Principles & Seven Practices.
(10) Use of the Samaritan method of active listening.
(11) Reliable daily service at specified times, aiming for 24 hour availability.

Finally, whilst being a Samaritan involves the giving of time, empathy and energy to those in distress, Samaritans everywhere say they in return receive more in terms of personal growth, awareness and fulfilment than they can ever give.

As the subject of this chapter is 'How to start a Branch', nothing has been said about the process by which a Probationary Branch is recognised as a full Branch of BI with representation on its governing councils, or about such a Branch's contribution towards the cost of maintaining BI.

Seven paces together is sufficient for the friendship of the virtuous, but thou and I have dwelt together.

THE VISHNU PURANA

Could I be a Samaritan?

The Samaritans have a continual need for part-time volunteers to help them maintain and expand the vital community service they offer.

We are looking for volunteers who feel they would be able to listen supportively and compassionately and to help anyone who is lonely, frightened, in trouble or has come to the point when they feel life is no longer worth living. If you are prepared to give up a little of your spare time, are able to see people's problems as greater than your own and, above all, are a good listener, you could well be the type of person for whom the Samaritans are looking.

Do I need any qualifications?
No. Samaritan volunteers come from all walks of life and anyone of any age, sex, social background, religion or race can apply.

How do I volunteer?
Write to the Branch or ring them and one of the volunteers on duty will be happy to tell you a little more about what is entailed.

What happens then?
You will probably be invited to come down into the local centre for a chat and if both you and the Samaritans decide it is suitable for you, you will be required to attend preparation classes with other trainee volunteers.

What training am I given?
We do not call it training because it is impossible to teach

anyone to listen warmly, sympathetically and patiently. Nor can you train people to be sensitive and pick up real feelings and thoughts.

Each Branch prepares its new volunteers in a slightly different way but you can be sure that you will be given a good insight into the work and your suitability for it before you are asked to befriend callers.

How much time must I give?

Once accepted for duty, a Samaritan volunteer is expected to do a regular 3-4 hour duty every week or in some Branches a slightly longer shift once a fortnight. These shifts usually include your fair share of overnight duties.

Where will I work?

All duties are done in the centre so you don't need your own car or telephone. And as we only use first names, you will never be put in the position of callers knowing your full name, address or telephone number.

What support am I given?

For the first few months, a new Samaritan will have regular meetings with a more experienced volunteer. After that, there are on-going training sessions and Branch meetings when volunteers meet to share their ideas. Regionally there is a regular programme of day and weekend training schools and conferences which volunteers may also attend.

The important difference between the most helpable callers and Samaritan volunteers is that the former are temporarily incapacitated by their neuroses whilst the latter are permanently made uneasy by theirs if they attempt to live for themselves alone.

ED.

On being a volunteer – NUALA KELLY

There are many unusual aspects to Samaritan life: aspects which can only be seen when one stands back after a couple of years and tries to look objectively at an organisation that has become a part of one's life. The most unusual aspect is the extraordinary ability of The Samaritans to enrol people who are active by nature, verbally and physically concerned for their fellow men, and to turn them into passive, compassionate listeners; to put in the background the very 'self' that first attracted the volunteers to this particular type of work.

Samaritans soon learn that the simple requirement of a listening ear carries with it many demands. The natural compassionate response to someone in distress has to be guided by a degree of detachment that leaves the volunteer free of emotive judgements and at the same time allows him to be emotionally concerned for the client.

The Samaritan does not need to be versed in psychiatry, psychology or the social services but he needs discipline . . . he must be prepared to feel inadequate and accept this blow to his ego. He has to trust his fellow volunteers to take over clients from him, fully confident that each one of them will be just as efficient as he is himself, sometimes even more so. He has to avoid pre-judgement, free advice, snap summing-up of problems; he has to accept that he is required to do some office-work so that the best service can be given to the client at all times. He has unfortunately to change the initial picture of himself sitting with phone in hand, his heart full of concern, his ear attuned to every nuance in his caller's voice and divine inspiration endowing him with just the right word at the right moment all the time. Divine inspiration and an ear well tuned-in we all need, but usually it is in retrospect that we realise the deficiencies of our contribution to conversations and we remember all too late some of the cardinal rules we learned in training.

Volunteers have to resist their natural impulse to solve some desperate cases by giving material comfort . . . they have to accept that a client's sworn promise to phone next day is often not kept . . . they have to accept that gratitude doesn't necessarily follow weeks and months of time spent on cases . . . that often the person helped doesn't even remember his name. The volunteer discovers that he is what he actually chose to be – faceless, nameless, just a voice or an ear and nothing more.

It is hard to be so anonymous, and often the volunteer's own personality refuses to accept such a low profile. The desire to build up problems, to over-emphasise situations or to decide without consultation that certain people seeking help are merely a nuisance, is very tempting. The volunteer has to accept that what appeared easy and natural to his personality demands greater effort and discipline, discernment, concern and self-effacement than at first realised.

The attraction of working as an individual under the umbrella of a recognised organisation still remains but the responsibilities this brings to the volunteer usually become apparent only after practical application of training. Volunteers meet other volunteers so they can't keep their concern only for the telephone or the consulting room, it has to encompass their fellow workers, the upkeep of the premises, the running of the organisation, the flag-days and the ongoing training programme that are all part and parcel of The Samaritans. Those who come seeking an outlet for their compassionate natures suddenly find themselves asked to do the very work that they had run from in other organisations. The Samaritans demands the essence – that great dichotomy between the active and the passive . . . it requires ordinary people to be extraordinary even if only for a few hours a fortnight.

It requires that people of diverse interests and backgrounds work together conscious that personalities often don't blend, and that the volunteers who take on far more than the normal work load need the co-operation of the others, or at least the understanding that what they are doing is an answer to one of the needs of the organisation and not just glory-seeking. The critical faculty which our training endeavours to eradicate for the benefit of our clients should not rear its head in the confines of the Centre and be directed to those who volunteer or who are asked to take on more onerous duties. Each one, no matter how elevated his position in the organisation, is still a Samaritan giving the full measure of the time and ability which he can afford to this voluntary work.

The clients create us; for them we exist. We have to refrain from the danger of creating ourselves into something superlative, in manipulating our clients just to boost our own ego – even if our clients very often manipulate us to their own advantage.

Je me regrette.

The young Vicomtesse d'Huededot at the guillotine.

Care of the volunteers – JOHN ELDRID*

Who cares for the volunteers?

For every Director of a Samaritan Branch this is a vital question as care of the volunteers is his responsibility. I emphasise *responsibility*, because it does not imply that the Director cares for all the volunteers personally, which is generally impossible and in many situations not beneficial; but the Director is responsible for seeing that the volunteers are cared for, by himself/herself, Deputy Directors, Leaders and any one else appointed for the job.

But before the Director can effectively be *responsible* for the care of volunteers, he/she must have appropriate care for himself or herself – and indeed have accepted his own personal need for care. The Lord says, '*Love your neighbour as yourself*'. This implies, first, that you know how to love yourself. How you do this is your personal business. You will need to recognise that the emotional, spiritual, sexual and social aspects all need attention and satisfaction. You may effectively be cared for by your wife, husband, friends, homosexual partner, or as part of a religious order, but I do not think the Director should expect to rely for total care on the members of the Branch.

I do not mean that volunteers should not and do not care for their Director. I am very much aware of the great care I have received from Portsmouth and London Branches. But there is a need for the Director to have loving, caring relationships outside the Branch. I recognise that working in The Samaritans may change one and enrich one's personal life and

* Talk given at a School for Leaders, Swanwick, March 1976.

relationships, but this is not the same thing as a total dependence on The Samaritans for a meaning to life. This also applies to volunteers though there are some differences, since the task of the Director is more demanding than that of a volunteer, so it is possible for volunteers to have a wider area of dependence for personal and social needs on The Samaritans than a Director can have. We come back to the Director's responsibility for care of volunteers. Let us first draw out the areas of concern and need, and secondly, suggest ways to meet our responsibility.

Areas of concern and need

Anxiety is one of the major problems for all of us. I would be so bold as to suggest that the only real problem in The Samaritans is the anxiety of the volunteers, and not necessarily the problems of the clients. If we can cope with our own anxiety, then we are likely to befriend our caller well. This means that volunteers, new and old, will want to have opportunities for talking about their anxieties regarding calls, outside befriending and so on. As we know, neurotic anxiety is the result of a situation of conflict. So if a volunteer feels anxious, it may be because the caller has triggered off some unresolved emotional conflict. No matter how carefully selected volunteers are, it is likely that at some time a caller will awaken some unresolved emotional problems in them. It is always rather a shock when the caller outlines his problems and difficulties and you find you have more or less the same difficulties!

From my experience in The Samaritans it would seem that on the whole volunteers cope quite well with bearing and sharing the distress of our callers, but the trouble comes when the caller touches or triggers off a neurotic fear, sexual problem, or pet hate. So when a volunteer seems unduly anxious about a caller, we may need to ask, 'What has the caller started off in the volunteer?' The volunteer's anxiety about the caller may be only the 'presenting problem'!

I am well aware that volunteers are remarkable and special people, but I am realistic enough to recognise we all come with mixed motives. From the evidence of a recent questionnaire, some of us are rather nervous about recognising that we have mixed motives for joining. Even after careful selection, the motives for seeking to reduce personal inner loneliness, or to gain power or the satisfaction of sexual curiosity, are still likely to be present. I know that most Directors, at some time or other, have experience of those who have not resolved their neurotic need for power. So we can in spite of careful selection expect to be troubled by some of these common feelings.

This means that often volunteers will need help to find ways of coping with and redirecting such motivations. We must be realistic about them and not be afraid to look at the so-called darker side of our personalities. We can thus help our volunteers to become more mature persons. Carl Rogers' little book called 'Encounter Groups' is well worth reading. Many Samaritans have experience of Encounter Group activities. I am not suggesting that Encounter Groups will give us all the answers, but his book and such group experience are worthy of our attention.

Some volunteers will find it hard to accept direction and guidance. They want to 'go it alone'. A lot of potentially good volunteers seem to have problems about Branch discipline, so we need to handle them with understanding.

We have to recognise that volunteers may become tired and lose – for a time, anyway – their ability to fulfil the emotional demands of our work. In many Branches, especially in the large cities, the pressure of work is very demanding. I am keenly aware of this in London. On the other hand, in less busy Branches volunteers may lose heart through not having enough to do.

The volunteer who is in contact, whether long term or short term, with a client who kills himself/herself, will feel very vulnerable for a time. I personally have been closely involved with a number of suicides and some of the emotional scars still remain. So we should expect such volunteers to have a bereavement period, often with a lot of guilt feelings which are not justified. Many of our volunteers have suffered from quite serious depression and I am not suggesting this affects their quality as volunteers, for any of us may be depressed, but we may attract people who are more likely to become more depressed and suicidal than the average person. I think it is worth bearing this in mind in the choice of volunteers.

How we carry out the responsibility for care of volunteers

I suggest there are five ways in which this responsibility may be carried out, by the Director, Deputy Directors and Leaders, Tutors to new volunteers, Groups and the Branch as a whole.

First, the Director is responsible for doing all he or she can to develop these five avenues of care. This kind of set-up presupposes the concept of a shared responsibility and leadership. So the Director, who knows that if he or she should die or move suddenly, Joe or Mary will take over, is already realistically caring for the volunteers.

I have already said it is impossible in a large Branch for the Director to care personally for all the volunteers, and it is probably unhealthy for this to happen in a small Branch where it *is* possible. I do, however, consider the Director should see all volunteers who are involved with a client who kills himself/herself. Special attention should also be given to volunteers who are involved with police or a court case. Quite apart from expert guidance, the volunteer may need a lot of befriending support.

Where volunteers have to be dismissed it is the Director's business to do it. We would hope all volunteers know the Director is available to talk with them about personal matters or serious Samaritan problems. At the same time, the fact that you are the Director may stop some volunteers from coming to you with personal problems, because the Director's first responsibility is to serve the clients, and also the Director is concerned with Branch discipline.

Secondly, most of us will have found that at least one Deputy Director or Leader will emerge as the confidant(e) of many volunteers. This can be most helpful, but it is better if this can be a shared responsibility. Deputy Directors and Leaders should be the kind of people who are able to care for volunteers as well as for clients. They can do much valuable work by being sensitive to the needs of volunteers who are emotionally upset by a client's problems. The attitude of the Deputy Directors and Leaders in general will of course very much reflect that of the Director. If the Director is able to share responsibility and care of the volunteers and indeed the whole Branch, then the Deputy Directors and Leaders are more likely to express their own special gifts of leadership and care. In this way the care of volunteers is able to develop naturally. How you organise and care for volunteers who are befriending callers outside the Centre depends on local Branch needs, but it is essential for volunteers to feel able to talk to Leaders about their anxieties regarding ongoing befriending. We have to recognise that some volunteers feel guilty about bothering the Director, Deputy Directors and Leaders, so they need encouragement. Expecting them to send in regular 'follow-up' reports is useful, and of course to report any worsening or improvement of the client's situation.

The third point concerns the 'Tutor System', especially for helpers. I suggest that when you become a helper you should automatically join a helpers' group and have your own tutor. This helps to reduce anxiety and gives the helpers opportunities to talk freely among themselves and with their tutor. It is very good if the helpers can meet at their tutor's home, but this is not always possible. In a large Branch it takes a while to get a tutor system going well, so a lot of patience and faith is needed. But it is extremely valuable in many ways, e.g. often it is through the care and counsel of a good tutor that a rather shy volunteer may blossom into a very confident Samaritan. The tutors also enable the Director to make a fairer assessment of a volunteer's suitability to become a Member. And of course helpers do seem to be very willing to bring their personal worries to their tutor.

The fourth way of caring is through groups. I am thinking especially of the building up of area groups of volunteers who live within a reasonable distance of each other. Such a group, with a Leader or other experienced Samaritan, has regular meetings during the year, usually once a month or every six weeks. The Director, Consultants, or others can be invited from time to time. The main business of the group of about twelve volunteers is to share their anxieties, befriend each other, and further their Samaritan education. Again you need a lot of patience in getting such groups going.

Lastly, there is the care given by the Branch as a whole. This is very important to develop and is much easier in a small Branch than in a large one. Some Branches have regular Branch meetings and I am sure this is beneficial, but we should always recognise that a lot of inter-communication between more than fifteen or so people is not really likely.

It is possible for a large Branch meeting to split into groups for a while, but the value of a Branch meeting is surely to experience the togetherness of the Branch and this can be expressed in social functions with some limited business. When possible I think it is good to be able to invite non-Samaritans, especially husbands, wives and so on, to socials, as there is a danger of volunteers becoming a kind of club.

As part of the care of volunteers the Branch should offer opportunities for on-going education and encourage the Branch to realise they are part of a great association of Branches.

The key points in the care of volunteers are lots of consultation, shared leadership, and firm direction.

Quis custodiet custodes? Who takes care of the caretakers?

Suicide in Hungary – BELA BUDA

Hungary's suicide situation is unique and puzzling. There is no other country in the world where such a marked and almost continuous rise in the number of suicidal deaths has taken place in the last two decades. Hungary's suicide rate was 26.0 per 100,000 per annum in 1960, 29.8 in 1965, 34.6 in 1970, 38.1 in 1975 and 44.9 in 1980. It is certain that this steady increase is real and cannot be attributed to changes in the identification of suicidal cases or in the statistical reporting system.

The suicide rate in Hungary has always been high. In the last hundred years at least, Hungary has always been among the nations with the highest suicide rates.

Foreign experts on suicidology frequently express the opinion that because of these two interesting features – the continuous increase of suicide cases on the one hand, and a high baseline rate on the other – Hungary would be an ideal field for research into suicide. Unfortunately Hungarians do not seem to share this opinion, because there is no tradition of suicide research in the country, funds are not available for it, nor is official support given. Except for five or six studies – all of these done in the last fifteen years – we have practically no research data which could illuminate the problem more clearly than the official statistics do. These statistics themselves, too, are rather difficult of access as they are published only in restricted circles. Suicide is a sort of 'skeleton in the cupboard' for the country, and not a proper topic to speak about, even among scientists. National pride and political uneasiness contribute to the neglect of the study of the manifestation and causes of suicide because the high rate has, for a long time, been thought to be a sign of the nation's biological or spiritual weakness, or a symptom of tension within the political system.

Owing to the scarcity of research data everything we know about suicide in Hungary is based on or deduced from the analysis and interpretation of statistical tables, generalisations from clinical material and case studies, impressions gained from folklore and history, or, at best, results of small scale investigations. Every explanation concerning suicide in Hungary is, therefore, of a hypothetical and theoretical character.

This must be said before exploring some questions and problems of our suicide scene in more detail. A series of observations points to the deduction that the constant high suicide rate in Hungary reflects the influence of Hungarian culture. Suicide is deeply ingrained in the Hungarian population: a form of culturally offered and condoned solution in situations where severe existential failure, loss of honour or of a beloved person, or a feeling of rejection and isolation is experienced. Public opinion stores up a wide array of *understandable* or *excusable* patterns of suicide, which are discussed in everyday talk – especially after suicides in the local community – with open or hidden approval or appreciation. Thus a complex set of values and norms is transmitted concerning suicide and this is a part of the socialisation process too. Attitudes and other elaborate cognitive schemes are formed which help people to define interpersonal situations (e.g. frustrations, conflicts, crimes, chronic or incapacitating illnesses, moral crimes, disappointments, etc.) as being intolerable and to be reacted to with a suicidal act, with escape through suicide following. Death is 'romanticised' in Hungarian folklore. Popular attitudes stress suicide as a proper expression of hatred and punishment against persons who are considered the immediate cause of an emotional crisis. So people kill themselves not only from exasperation and wish to escape from an impossible life situation, but also to strike a blow at somebody, to elicit guilt feelings in somebody.

Our popular culture is prone to let persons who are in trouble be isolated and victimised. Such people know from their own experience what to expect from others in the case of serious problems. Sometimes this contributes to the motivation of suicide, both in the form of escape-seeking and of a wish for a hateful revenge.

The role of the cultural factor is shown in the fact that the high suicide rate in Hungary is found also amongst the Hungarian populations over the borders in neighbouring countries. It may also be noted that Hungarian ethnic groups in countries overseas have high suicide rates. Another remarkable fact is the territorial difference in suicide rates between different parts of the country. The suicide rate is about 50% higher in the south-eastern parts than in the western or north-western areas. The distribution of different suicide rates is stable and patterned, and cannot be explained by religion, age structure or socio-economic circumstances. Explanations of the differences between different parts of the country rely on the assumption that there must be differences between regional sub-cultures concerning *suicidality*. Culture as an explanatory principle can be used in other ways too: for instance, if we suppose that culture not only regulates proneness to commit suicide but also the degree or quantity of life stresses or the probability of a person suffering a depressive illness. We don't have any data about the mediating role of depression between culture and suicide although this role cannot be excluded. Culture may have *depressiogenic* characteristics: it may regulate alcohol consumption and alcohol abuse, which we know to be a factor in influencing the number of suicides. Unfortunately, we have only suppositions about this problem in relation to Hungary. This is also relevant to the increase of suicidal deaths in Hungary in the last few decades. The possibility cannot be excluded that the rapid rise in alcohol consumption, the growing number of known alcoholics and the somatic and psychiatric complications of chronic alcoholism help to determine the increase of suicides. Alcohol consumption and alcoholism, however, spread much more widely and in a higher degree than suicide. A circumstance weighing against the etiological role of depression is that the prescription of antidepressant drugs is increasing by geometrical progression in Hungary, even in general practice, and Hungarian doctors adopt a very broad diagnostic category of depression, in consequence of which a lot of people are labelled *'masked' depressive*. In addition, the use of lithium prophylaxis is growing. Nevertheless, the number of suicidal deaths and of the known cases of suicidal attempts increases. Not even the constantly improving somatic care of the suicidal 'attempters' in emergency units can counteract the increase of suicidal deaths. This shows that a biological explanation of suicide frequency is rather difficult to hold, especially taking into consideration the continuous increase found in Hungary.

The true explanation of the Hungarian rise in suicides seems to lie on the sociological or socio-psychological level. Hungary's rising suicide rate represents a typical example of Durkheim's *anomie theory*. The rising trend of suicide goes parallel with the growing prosperity and affluence of the Hungarian population, and with the growing social freedom of the individual. The mediating variables are industrialisation and urbanisation, connected with an unprecedented vertical and horizontal mobility. A very high proportion of the population has changed its occupation, domicile and former life style, moving mostly to big cities and industrial areas. The dissolution of the traditional communities has brought about secularisation, even in the Roman Catholic part of the population. The rise of alcohol consumption is connected with the socio-economic expansion of the society. The habit of competition has arisen in practically all spheres of life. Individual self-fulfilment and the attainment of the dominant material values have become the chief goals for people. This may be called *anomie* – a state of societal and interpersonal affairs which makes the use of former orientation schemes difficult, and which is liable to disorient people, e.g. by forcing them to choose new comparative and normative reference groups for themselves, by discouraging them from seeking help from strangers in their new communities, and by inciting competitive impulses in them without a real necessity for competition. This state of affairs is placing heavy burdens on some groups or social categories, e.g. on the older people, on the deviant and on the disadvantaged. The old particularly are considered a nuisance to their family when it is taking part in competitive striving towards the dominant values. Marriage and family life is adversely affected too, as is manifested in the increase in the number of divorces (a very clear trend in today's Hungary) and the children brought up without one of the parents.

Anomie then causes many personal problems and conflicts – anxieties, damage to self-esteem, frustrations because of intensification of some desires and expectations – and these are expressed in the form of the sick role, in psychiatric illness or substance-abusive behaviour. All this increases the probability of suicidal behaviour. The personal crisis reinforces the hidden behaviour patterns of suicide learned in the socialisation process.

The Hungarian suicide statistics show that the increase in the number of suicidal deaths mostly manifests itself in the elevated frequency of self-destruction among older people, the growth being higher among older women. Women's suicides are increasing in all age categories. There is also a rapid increase in the suicide of middle-aged men (this can be brought into connection with alcoholism). Equally, there is a marked increase among married men and those living in families. Marriage and family conflicts, as well as isolation and rejection, are in clear relationship with a considerable number of suicides. All these manifestations may be signs of a societal process which is similar to that described by Durkheim under the concept of *anomie*.

It has been observed in Hungary that a very large number of suicides visited their doctors before committing the self-destructive act. A big group of suicidal persons had been to psychiatrists and obtained some diagnostic labels and some treatment. Contact with doctors seems to be obviously inefficient in preventing suicide. A lot of circumstances make the assumption not too far-fetched that an important part of the increase in the number of suicidal deaths is played also by inadequacy of the present-day psychiatric and social-supportive service system in Hungary. There are not enough facilities for outpatient psychiatric care. Up to now there are no units of crisis intervention, only plans to organise such units. General practitioners and somatic specialists lack training, interest, knowledge and time to detect and solve suicidal crises. Serious cases are sent to psychiatrists who are trained only in traditional psychiatric nosology or in biological psychiatry, and who have only two choices: either to label the patient a depressive and give him drugs, or send him to a locked ward for protection against the danger of suicide. The pre-suicidal syndrome is frequently overlooked, and most Hungarian doctors don't even know the concept, let alone possess the capability of differentiating this psychodynamic state of personality from a depression in cases when the two states do not go together. There is no occupation which would correspond to the speciality of the social worker. Only a few clinical psychologists now work in the field of suicide prevention. The suicidal patient will not usually receive psychological help or a properly supporting physician-patient relationship from doctors. Lack of research in suicidology and scarcity of interest in phenomena of suicide in medical and scientific circles are then coupled with an inadequate psychological attitude and lack of empathy and readiness to help with psychotherapeutic methods. This circumstance may play a role in the high suicide rate, and is the reverse of the situation in Britain, where leading suicide researchers hold the opinion that a better training of general practitioners and other doctors in suicidology, and improved secondary and tertiary care are an important factor in the decrease of suicidal deaths.

The fact remains that Hungary would be an interesting field of suicide research and a suitable testing ground of the effectiveness of different methods of suicide prevention. We can only hope that in the next few years the health authorities and the representatives of social sciences will realise the severity and, at the same time, the scientific interest of our suicidal situation and will begin supporting research and prevention.

When they told me you were gone
I remembered how the sun,
Heraclitus, time and again
Set on our talks; and I wept then.
Halicarnassus saw you born.
Somewhere dust now picks your bone.
But though Death takes everything
Your 'Nightingales' still sing, ah sing!

CALLIMACHUS

The Samaritans: plan for a school

One of the most valuable features of Samaritan work in the British Isles has been the series of Schools held at Swanwick in Derbyshire, for Directors, for Leaders, for Publicity Officers and Fund-raisers. Experience shows that some kind of a plan is essential, and the following one (devised in 1979) was organised in three 'modules', each consisting of a plenary or demi-plenary, a workshop and the chance to talk out issues raised (or anything else) in small groups.

(Module A – The Opening Plenary)

Befriending and the community

Evidence suggests that we permeate the community indirectly and directly – *indirectly* in that it is known that The Samaritans are always there and available, even if not used – a sort of talisman. We are known through publicity, professional links and the grapevine, also through recruitment and fund-raising which is also publicity. This awareness leads to a sense of dependence and security that something precious is being preserved.

But *directly*, how far have we managed to put suicide on the agenda of public and professional concern? How far does the public really understand the nature and limitations of our work? What is the proper response to their expectations and trust?

'Talisman: Anything that acts as a charm or by which extra-ordinary results are achieved. 1784.' (*Shorter O.E.D.*, 1972.)

(Extra Demi-plenary)

Society, suicide and The Samaritans over the last and the next thirty years
Having passed our thirty-third anniversary, it is appropriate to look back at the changes in society since we began – probably greater than in any equivalent period – especially in relation to suicide, confidentiality, the law, the family, corporatism, attitudes to authority, attitudes between the generations, expectations of relationships.

Also there is a need to try to anticipate the next few years, for change will continue. Are we able to meet emerging needs? Are we a movement or an institution?

'The Samaritans simply lacked the way of adjusting to novel situations'.

(*The Scientific American*, January, 1977.)

Befriending and the community (Workshops)
(Workshop A 1)
Liaison with local professional and voluntary agencies
'Your branch is lucky, we have no consultants.'

'Surely we've outgrown consultants – don't need to depend on professionals.'

'What do Samaritans do anyway? Shouldn't we discourage them from meddling with this patient of ours?'

'There is a need for a new sort of service halfway between a Citizen's Advice Bureau and a crisis centre, staffed by volunteers where people can go when . . .' (Evidence of the Conference of Chief Probation Officers *Marriage Matters*, Home Office 1978).

'The Samaritans represent an extreme in isolationism . . .' (*The Scientific American*, January 1977).

In this workshop, participants will meet with a consultant psychiatrist, a social worker and a general practitioner and will explore how healthy are our relationships with our friends with whom we share the care of our callers.

(Workshop A 2)
Getting the message across
This workshop stresses the commitment of leaders (and all

members) to the general policy of the Branch. Publicity affects the potential clients and volunteers who do or do not approach us. The way in which we treat clients and others who have occasion to ring us is the principal means of publicity and cannot but do good or harm. So does even the style of fund-raising and the content and manner of talks.

But to most of us the media represent not a means of publicity but a threatening intrusion on the cosy life of the Branch. So let's have a look at it.

'The media is a whore. Screw it – or you'll get screwed by it.' (Anon. journalist, 1979).

(Workshop A 3)
Getting the right people, or making a match
In this workshop we consider the nature of the attachment between the volunteer and Samaritan (Branch) work. The framework chosen as illustration is that of a marriage or close friendship and the purpose is to raise the kind of questions which members can readily apply to their own Branches. The essential relationship is *mutual compatibility* rather than one partner 'selecting' the other. The sub-headings we shall use are – Early Initiatives, A Developing Relationship, Living Together, The Parting of the Ways.

'Getting to know you,
Getting to know all about you;
Getting to like you,
Getting to hope *you* like *me*!' (O. Hammerstein II)

(Workshop A 4)
Public relations and fund-raising
This workshop examines the ethics and the publicity involved in attracting funds. While many members do not *have* to fund-raise, they should, as part of their commitment to the Branch, be aware of the Samaritan implications of fund-raising and all that goes with it. What means should we not use? Are some Friends failed Samaritans? They still represent and speak for the Branch. Does the Branch budget get

published to the Branch? Does it provide for all it should? What about the Annual Report?

> 'The naughtiness of the silver.' (Bishop Latimer on a previous bout of inflation.)

'Yes, but don't forget a billion dollars doesn't go as far as it used to.'
(The late Paul Getty)

(Workshop A 5)
Anonymity
If a caller exercises his or her right to remain unnamed, does it hinder befriending? Do we press too hard for the name sometimes? Are we more anxious to fit the 'case' into the Branch's experience (index system) than to establish a relationship at the caller's desired level?

Anonymity is our defence from too close an attachment by the caller. It is also a safeguard against the seeker after public acclaim who is attracted to voluntary work. But does it hinder real befriending? And is the effort of the volunteer in avoiding discovery of their Samaritan involvement really necessary?

'But still keep something to yoursel'
Ye scarcely tell to ony.'
(*Epistle to a Young Friend*, Robert Burns)

(Module B: Demi-plenary)

Befriending the individual *(Workshops)*
This session concentrates on our work with individual callers. 'Befriending' is the word we use to describe the relationship with all callers from the beginning and also the one-to-one relationship set up in cases of ongoing need. It needs to be distinguished from ordinary friendship: what are the distinctions? Can a Branch be said to 'befriend' in any recognisable sense of the word? Doesn't this deny the need for real one-to-one relationships for lack of which the callers come to us? Or are we talking about counselling anyway? What about advice-giving and problem-solving? We deny them and yet answer the phone 'The Samaritans. Can I help you?' when we mean 'The Samaritans. Can you help yourself?'

> 'He had probably never set himself up to understand . . . he had been content to play the holy humble role of service . . . to provide the sound of his voice to distract me from the crying of the silence.'
>
> (*The Waterfall*, Margaret Drabble)

(Workshop B 1)
Monitoring 'companioning' (assigned befriending)
This workshop concentrates on the leaders' role in helping 'companioning', i.e. befriending assigned to individual Samaritans meeting individual callers away from the Centre. Are they briefed on what is expected of them and warned of possible dangers? Sample role-plays may show the setting up of a companioning relationship, a befriender becoming possessive of his/her client, and the switching or termination of a companioning. What are the criteria for this latter? Do we appreciate the client's reaction to a switch or switching off? Are we prepared for the befriender's sense of loss, or resentment of the Leader's need to probe what's going on?

> 'Oh, do not ask, "What is it?"
> Let us go and make our visit!'
>
> (*The Love Song of Alfred J. Prufrock*, T. S. Eliot)

(Workshop B 2)
Befriending the elderly
This workshop will ask, What is the attitude of society to the elderly? Are there new problems that the elderly did not face in past generations? It will point to the intensification of loneliness through deafness and immobility, the sense of running downhill and being useless. Is current propaganda for euthanasia adding to this? Ought the Samaritans to become an adoptive family? Or one's Samaritan an adopted daughter? The problems posed by some old people's irrational pride. The extent to which we can and should liaise with other agencies. The valuable contribution of the old in befriending (inside and outside Samaritan work). Sample role-plays could include the lady who is very neglected but won't accept help for fear of having to be put away in the asylum, and the exhausting repetition of an old person's conversation.

(Workshop B 3)
Befriending the young
Our publicity is doing much to attract the young – do we know how to cope with them when they phone or visit? The workshop examines the difficulties, such as the tendency to exhibit parental reflexes – anxiety, problem-solving, 'talk to your parents/teacher,' 'you ought to be home by now, they'll be worried about you'. The question of matching young callers with young volunteers – is it always right? Can we listen directly to a mid-teens client without all sorts of luggage getting in the way? What about 'hoax' or testing calls?

We have more young volunteers in some branches than in others. Can our attitudes to young volunteers be the touchstone for our attitudes to young callers? Does the Branch welcome and use a student who is a Samaritan at college elsewhere?

> 'So many ways to be unsure or bold.'
> (*The Young Ones*, Elizabeth Jennings)

(Workshop B 4)
Befriending the addicted, or Smack, booze and us
This workshop examines and endeavours to make clear to members the main addictions and how we may be affected by them; and what help it is possible for us to give. It considers especially the problems that may lie behind the addiction; our relations with other agencies; and our care as Leaders for those befriending the addicted.

Why do addicts not contact us more? Are we perhaps frightened of addiction?

> 'Every form of addiction is bad, no matter whether to Narcotics, Alcohol, Morphine or Idealism.'
> (C. G. Jung.)

(Workshop B 5)
Befriending the befriender
This workshop tries to work out the best ways of supporting the befrienders of our callers and to look at their various sources of support when their companioning or 'one-off'

befriending contacts leave them with a sense of strain and failure (or indeed ought to and don't).

> 'I politely answered, but after a while I could detect in his voice the same note that I could hear in my own – a note of diffident, hopeless, anxious concern, striving with immense effort to sound detached and unconcerned. I felt so sorry for him, poor useless man, I knew that he was like me, equally afflicted and that that was why he was there on the end of that line at one o'clock in the morning, and I did not want him to know how irrelevant his questions were and how inexpressible my true complaints, so I tried hard to sound more cheerful to cheer him up so that he could ring off thinking that he had done a good job with me.'
>
> (*The Waterfall*, Margaret Drabble)

(Module C: Demi-plenary)

The boundaries of befriending

How far have the frontiers of Samaritan work been extended in recent years, and what have been the pros and cons? How far can they be extended in the future without breaching basic Samaritan principles? With the use of duos, trios, small groups and open discussion, this Demi-plenary session will begin to examine some vital areas, including training, support, accessibility and 'specialisation'. Have we tended to diversify because of the seeming success of our work shown in a reduced suicide rate, and are we now in need of rediscovering our original calling?

> 'Old men ought to be explorers.' (T. S. Eliot.)

(Workshop C 1)
Where and how do we draw the line?
The Boundaries of Befriending – which clients are unhelpable? Which might be harmed by befriending? What are the criteria? What are the priorities? How does this assessment affect the caller? . . . the volunteer? . . . the leader?

'If you want a client very well befriended, just put up a notice forbidding it.'

(Anon. Director to another, *c*. 1973.)

(Workshop C 2)
Samaritan Branches befriending in the open: The Festival Branch shares its experience
Since 1973 the Festival Branch has been befriending clients at pop and folk festivals, and other events. We have found that the way in which we work varies in some important aspects from that of static Branches. In this workshop we share what we have experienced and look at ways in which other Branches might learn from this and get involved in similar work.

'I couldn't help thinking of cosy Branches, and warm clean Centres, with the phone between you and the client. Here they came and you were face to face, and they could see your eyes and feel your hands, and you couldn't lounge back in the swivel chair and sip your coffee. I was sitting in the open with a distraught girl in floods of tears, and I held her hand, and she talked and talked. Will she visit her local Branch and accept befriending there too? I don't know – but here at Blackbush we were a crisis organisation, and isn't that what "Sams" is all about?'

(Volunteer attending her first Festival.)

(Workshop C 3)
The third party call
In June 1976 the Council resolved that we could respond much more to Third Party calls than before. This workshop explores the difficulties in deciding how to respond to differing types of call and then in either making an approach to the named person or in refusing to do so.

The workshop also considers who are the 'gatekeepers' who should know about our befriending and availability, e.g. policemen, night porters, chemists, caretakers, porters, bus conductors . . .

'Could you come and do something about our Alice? She was out until 9.30 *again* last night and she's only twenty-seven.'

(Anon. caller)

(Workshop C 4)
Bigger is better or small is beautiful? What sort of Branches do we want?
There have been changes in the pattern of coverage, e.g. fewer new Branches are being formed and more sub-groups (but not many). Some sub-groups have stopped manning for lack of business. This workshop is not so much to advocate policy as to explore the advantages and disadvantages of working as volunteer and leader in the very busy Branch or in the very quiet sub-group – the problems of giving supervision, guidance and support, and the problems of morale. What are the likely changes in e.g. telecommunications and advertising?

'Not too little, not too much, but just right.'
(The classic advertisement for Erasmic.)

(Workshop C 5)
What are the lessons and limits of Brenda?
The workshop explores the question of the Sexually Demanding Caller as a problem for Branches with a Brenda system and without one, especially as experienced by a male or female Leader responsible for female volunteers taking such calls. The problems that occur in referring such callers from a Branch without Brenda to a Branch with Brenda.

'But are they all horrid, are you sure they are all horrid?'
Catharine Morland in Jane Austen's *Northanger Abbey*

One-ended Role Play – A BRENDA

As only Brendas normally hear Brenda callers, it is difficult to get male Samaritans to play convincingly the role of a Brenda caller when using role play for instructional purposes. Chad therefore invented the One-ended Role Play especially for his pet Brendas, in Malaysia, Portugal, Brazil, London, etc.

In reading the following, you have to imagine that you are sitting with Brenda while she takes a call and can hear what she says but not what the caller says, which you have to deduce from her responses.

Brenda: Yes, who is that? . . . *Colin!*? Did you say 'Colin'? . . . Am I supposed to know you? . . . Yes, this is Brenda . . . No, I'm not a new one, and if I were, I'd know all the accepted callers . . . Oh, *you're* a new one? So how did you get this number? . . . I see. Well, what do you want, Colin – if that's your name? . . . You want to wank? Well, you don't have to have *my* permission. Wank away . . . Your friend told you I'd talk sexy to you to make it more exciting, did he? Well, he was wrong. Wank yourself silly, for all I care, but I'm not going to feed you your favourite fantasies while you do so . . . What do you mean, 'before'? You said you were a new caller . . . Well, Harry, I think the moment has come to tell you that I recognise your voice, and furthermore, that I know why you are pretending to be someone else . . . Look, you can either be Colin, and I shall replace the receiver at once, or you can be Harry, in which case we will continue the conversation for a while . . . Hello, Harry. You've got something you specially want to say to Brenda, haven't you? . . . An apology, Harry . . . I think you know, Harry, but if you prefer *me* to tell *you*, I will . . . OK, Harry – yesterday you committed the unforgivable sin . . . Don't talk daft, Harry, masturbation isn't a sin at all, let alone an unforgivable one. But what you did was something that Brenda will not tolerate . . . As if you didn't know, I'll tell you; yesterday you told Brenda you were desperate, and instead of having a friendly conversation with her first, you begged her to tell you your favourite fantasy of the platinum blonde with the muscular bottom, promising that you would have a really lovely chat afterwards. But then, you stinker, as soon as you'd come, you hung up . . . Oh yes you did . . . No, it wasn't two other fellows, it was you . . . No, there was no technological malfunction of the apparatus. You treated her like *dirt*, Harry, and you are now crossed off our list . . . Look, Harry, Brenda is a human being, a Samaritan, trying to befriend you, and she will not be treated like a mere convenience or a gramophone record. You are finished, Harry, and it's no good your ringing again, ever . . . Oh, you're sorry, are you? My guess is, you aren't sorry you treated Brenda like that, you're just sorry that you are going to suffer the consequences . . . Which Brenda am I? What difference does it make? We all take the same line. If it's any interest to you, I'm the 75-year-old nymphomaniac who earns her living as a fat woman in the circus . . . Yes, I know that's what Brenda said to you yesterday – I've just been reading it from her notes. Well now, will you hang up, or shall I? . . . What's that? You want me to plead with Brenda to give you another chance? Even if I thought you deserved it, what could I say? . . . Well, well – you surprise me, Harry. I didn't think you had it in you. OK, we will have *now* the conversation you should have had yesterday with Brenda, and I will report that you are truly penitent and solemnly promise never to do such a nasty thing again. What part of London do you live in? . . . Who else lives in the same house? . . . Older or younger than you? . . . What's your job? . . . *Ever* had one? . . . Why did you lose it? . . . What do you like doing, to pass the time? . . . Yes, I asked for that one, didn't I? I mean, besides wanking? . . . They've been playing quite well lately, haven't they? Who do you go with? . . . *Colin*! I might have known. How old is he? . . . Did you both go to the same school? . . . What school was that? . . . Was there anything you liked at school? . . . Really? What was *her* name? . . . Well, if Brenda agrees to accept your grovelling apology and put you back on the list,

I'll rehearse you in a few things you could say to that girl that might make her want to renew the acquaintance . . . Not at all, it'll be a pleasure . . . *What*!? What was that you said? . . . I hoped my old ears had deceived me. After all that's happened, you have the nerve to ask if you can wank *now*? . . . All right, I'll forget you said it . . . Yes, you can ring next Monday for the verdict – and mind you give your right name . . . Goodbye, Harry.

Between 1 January and 31 December 1985 Brenda recorded 1485 calls, equivalent to 123 a month or 5 a day. Half the callers were recognised as masturbating during the call. 79% of callers were single, 75% were blue collar workers or unemployed, 53% were aged between 20 and 30. The youngest caller was 13, the oldest 64. 22.5% were listed as 'persistent callers'. Several calls came from the USA.

Brenda Log Books

List of Branches of The Samaritans

This list gives the addresses and telephone numbers of all recognised Branches of The Samaritans (i.e. in the British Isles) and of Befrienders International (The Samaritans Worldwide) (i.e. everywhere in the world except the British Isles) committed to the Seven Principles and Seven Practices (see p. 71).

All the Branches of The Samaritans, whether in the United Kingdom, the Channel Islands, the Isle of Man or the Republic of Ireland, have their Branch number (which indicates their seniority) followed by /1. All are addressed as The Samaritans. They have been listed under the place where the Branch premises are situated, to make it easier for prospective callers. If the title of the Branch is different, its chosen title is given in brackets, e.g. The Samaritans of the Chilterns are listed under Amersham. Branches of The Samaritans are administered from 17 Uxbridge Road, Slough, SL1 1SN (tel. 0753 32713). The General Secretary is the Revd David Evans, MA, his Assistant is Mr Simon Armson, and the Administrative Officer is Mrs Vera Feeney.

Branches of Befrienders International (The Samaritans Worldwide) have their Branch number followed by a number from 2 to 46, according to the following code:

2 = Hong Kong	The Samaritans
3 = India	The Samaritans; & Helping Hand
4 = Zimbabwe	The Samaritans
5 = Pakistan	(The Samaritans)
6 = New Zealand	The Samaritans; & Life Link
7 = Australia	The Samaritans; & Life Link

8 = Poland	Anonimowy Przyjaciel
9 = Brazil	CVV-Samaritans: & Amigos Anônimos
10 = Singapore	(The Samaritans)
11 = Malaysia	The Befrienders
12 = USA	The Samaritans
13 = Republic of South Africa	The Samaritans – Die Samaritane
14 = Zambia	(The Samaritans)
15 = Sri Lanka	Sumithrayo
16 = France	S.O.S. Help
17 = Spain	(Amigos Internacionales)
18 = Sweden	Någon att tala med, Samaritans
19 = Austria	The Befrienders
20 = Mauritius	(The Samaritans)
21 = Argentina	CVV-Samaritanos
22 = Trinidad and Tobago	Lifeline – The Befrienders
23 = Colombia	CVV-Samaritanos
24 = Uruguay	CVV-Samaritanos
25 = Japan	Suicide Prevention Center
26 = Thailand	The Samaritans
27 = Surinam	(De Samaritanen)
28 = Egypt	(The Befrienders)
29 = Barbados	The Samaritans
30 = Portugal	Telefone da Amizade
31 = Vanuatu	(The Samaritans)
32 = Italy	The Samaritans
33 = Chile	(CVV-Samaritanos)
34 = Fiji	(The Samaritans)
35 = Kuwait	(The Samaritans)
36 = Canada	The Samaritans
37 = Mexico	Los Samaritanos
38 = Bahrain	The Befrienders
39 = Dubai	(The Befrienders)
40 = Venezuela	(CVV-Samaritanos)
41 = Korea	Love-Line
42 = Indonesia	Hotline Service Bersama
43 = Nigeria	(The Samaritans)
44 = Oman	The Befrienders

45 = The Philippines (The Samaritans)
46 = Kenya (The Samaritans)

Services in brackets are in preparation or abeyance.

Befrienders International (The Samaritans Worldwide) separated its administration from that of The Samaritans in 1974 in order to strengthen the weaker countries and spread more rapidly throughout the world. Its Founder-President, Chad Varah, served three terms of three years as Chairman, and was replaced as Chairman on 2 November 1983 by Mrs Vanda Scott, PO Box 50029, Dallas, TX75250, USA, to whom all official communications regarding Befrienders International (The Samaritans Worldwide) should now be addressed. From 1974 to 1983 Befrienders International was a Charitable Association registered under the laws of Switzerland, but in 1984 began to be registered in each of the relevant countries including the UK where its Commissioners' number is 326693 and its Company number is 1921053.

NB When writing to British Branches DO NOT PUNCTUATE THE POSTCODE.

The dialling codes given are those from London and other distant places; from nearby places substitute the code given in the local code-book.

6/1 **Aberdeen**, 60 Dee Street, AB1 2DS 0224 574488/9

163/1 **Aberystwyth** (Dyfed), 5 Trinity Road, SY23 1LU 0970 4535

1/9 **Abolição**-São Paulo, SP, Brazil, CVV-Samaritanos, Rua Abolíção 411, CEP 01319 011 34 4141

11/12 **Albany**, NY, USA. 200 Central Avenue NY 12203 (The Samaritans of the Capital District) 518 463 2323

5/7 **Albany**, Western Australia, 6330, POB 991 098 414777

33/9 **Americana**, SP, Brazil, CVV-Samaritanos, Rua 7 de Setembro 1000, CEP 13470 0194 610716

93/1 **Amersham**, 149 Station Road, HP6 6LZ (The Samaritans of the Chilterns) 02403 5000 & 21222

21/9 **Araçatuba**, SP, Brazil, CVV-Samaritanos, Rua Tabajaras 772, CEP 16100 0186 234111

24/9 **Araraquara**, SP, Brazil, CVV Samaritanos, Rua Gonçalves Diaz 1411, & Caixa Postal 314 CEP 14800 0162 364111

133/1 **Ashford**, 20 Queen Street, TN23 1RP 0233 24606/7

169/1 **Ashington**, 25 North Seaton Road, NE63 0AG 0670 814222

AYRSHIRE – see Kilmarnock

1/38 **Bahrain**, Arabian Gulf, The Befrienders, POB 1, Manama 276 222

155/1 **Ballymena**, 45 Mount Street, BT43 6BP 0266 58333/4

175/1 **Banbury**, 29a Albert Street, OX16 8DG 0295 57575

5/3 **Bangalore** 560001, India, Helping Hand, 9/1 Museum Road 577 188

1/26 **Bangkok 5**, Thailand, Christ Church, 11 Convent Road, POB 1220, B. 10501 235 4000/1

181/1 **Bangor**, Gwynedd, 7 Abbey Road LL57 2EA 0248 354 646

143/1 **Bangor**, 92 Dufferin Avenue, BT20 3AD (The Samaritans of Bangor & North Down) 0247 464646

1/29 **Barbados**, W. I., The Samaritans, Crelow, Strathclyde Crescent & POB 328, Bridgetown 427 0103

115/1 **Barnsley**, 11 Victoria Road, S70 2BB 0226 20222

88/1 **Barnstaple**, 2 Summerland Street, EX32 8JJ (The Samaritans of North Devon) 0271 74343

8/9 **Barra Funda**, São Paulo, SP, Brazil, CVV-Samaritanos, Rua Vitorino Carmilo 717, Anexo ao Pronto Socorro, CEP 01153 011 826 1025

52/9 **Barretos**, SP, Brazil, CVV-Samaritanos, Rua Doze 911 CEP 14780 0173 224 966

121/1 **Barrow**, 16 Hartington Street, LA14 5SL (The Samaritans of Furness) 0229 25656

87/1 **Basildon**, 16 Little Lullaway, SS15 5JJ (The Samaritans of Basildon & Thurrock) 0268 412000

139/1 **Basingstoke**, 5 Essex Road, RG21 1TA 0256 462333/4

52/1 **Bath**, 2 New King Street, BA1 2BL 0225 29222

30/9 **Baurú**, SP, Brazil, CVV-Samaritanos, Rua Batista de Cavalho 4-33. 6 sala 607, CEP 17100 0142 254 2551

37/1 **Bedford**, 69 Gwyn Street, MK40 1HH 0234 211211

17/9 **Belém**, PA, Brazil, CVV-Samaritanos, Travessa 1 de Marco 241, Sala 106, CEP 66000 091 2244141

13/1 **Belfast**, Thomson House, 46/48 Stranmillis Road, BT9 5AD 0232 664422

7/9 **Belo Horizonte**, MG, Brazil, CVV-Samaritanos, Rua Guaranesia 164, Floresta, CEP 30000 031 444 4141

174/1 **Bexleyheath**, 35 Glynde Road (The Samaritans of Bexley & Dartford) 301 1010

55/9 **Birigui**, SP, Brazil, CVV-Samaritanos, Rua Bento da Cruz 233 Centro, CEP 16200 0186 42 1910

25/1 **Birmingham**, 3 Brasshouse Passage, Broad Street, B1 2HR 021 643 8001

105/1 **Blackburn**, 105 New Park Street, BB2 1DF (The Samaritans of Blackburn, Hyndburn and Ribble Valley) 0254 662424

171/1 **Blackpool**, 16 Edward Street, FY1 1BA 0253 22218

1/13 **Bloemfontein, O.F.S.**, 9300 Republic of South Africa, Room 18, First Floor, Waldorf Bldg, Cnr, Maitland & President Brand Streets, and POB 2201 051 83000

BLOOMFIELD – see Hartford

118/1 **Bognor Regis**, 13 Argyle Road, PO21 1DY 0243 826333/4

68/1 **Bolton**, 16 Bark Street, BL1 2BQ 0204 21200

1/3 **Bombay 400008**, India, Seva Niketan, Sir J. Jeejibhai Road, Byculla 379846

BORDERS – see Selkirk

74A/1 **Boston**, Lincs., 52 Wormgate, PE21 6NS (Associate Group of Lincoln q.v.) 0205 66111

1/12 **Boston**, MA, USA, 500 Commonwealth Avenue, MA 02215 617 247 0220

9/1 **Bournemouth**, Blue Pillars, Upper Terrace Road, BH2 5NW (The Samaritans of Mid-Wessex) 0202 21999

168/1 **Bracknell**, 'Trevaughan', Easthampstead Road RG12 1NN 0344 55555/6

15/1 **Bradford**, 21 Marlborough Road, Manningham, BD8 7LD 0274 494949/0

22/9 **Bragança Paulista**, SP, Brazil, CVV-Samaritanos, Rua Dr Antonio da Cruz 484A, CEP 12900 011 433 4077

14/9 **Brasilia**, DF, Brazil, CVV-Samaritanos, SQS-Edifico Venancio IV, sala 311, Setor de Diversoes-Sul, CEP 70.300 061 225 8885 & 8830

82/1 **Brent**, London, 7 Meyrick Road, NW10 2EL 459 8585

173/1 **Bridgend**, 2 Green Street, Bridgend, Mid Glamorgan CF31 1HF 0656 62333

BRIDGETOWN – see Barbados

14A/1 **Bridlington**, Rear of Half Moon Hotel, North Street, YO15 2DZ (Associate Group of Hull, q.v.) 02626 71717

137/1 **Brierley Hill**, Hill Street, DY5 2UE 0384 78111

99/1 **Brighton**, 102 Clarendon Road, Hove, BN3 3WQ (The Samaritans of Brighton, Hove & District) 0273 772277

48/1 **Bristol**, 37 St Nicholas Street, BS1 1TP 0272 298787 (3 lines)

2/23 BUCARAMANGA, Colombia – in abeyance

2/4 **Bulawayo**, Zimbabwe, POB 806 65000

BURNLEY – see Pendle

182/1 **Bury**, 12 Tenterden Street, BL9 0EG 061 764 0055

131/1 **Bury St Edmunds**, 46 Well Street, IP33 1EQ 0284 2345

80A/1 **Buxton**, 1A Crescent View, Hall Bank, SK17 6EN 0298 6000

1/28 CAIRO, Egypt – temporarily in abeyance

CAITHNESS – see Thurso

2/3 **Calcutta** 700016, India, Flat 13, 53B Elliot Road 298 609

23/1 **Cambridge**, 1 Parker Street, CB1 1JL 0223 64455/6

32/9 **Campinas**, SP, Brazil, Suicide Prevention Centre, Rua Marechal Deodoro 1221, Centro, CEP 13.100 0192 31 4141

103/1 **Canterbury**, 14 Ivy Lane, CT1 1TU 0227 457777

CAPE COD – see Falmouth

72/1 **Cardiff**, 75 Cowbridge Road East, Canton, CF1 9AF 0222 44022

112/1 **Carlisle**, 12 Corporation Road, CA3 8XB 0228 44444

CENTRAL LONDON BRANCH – see London

CENTRAL SCOTLAND – see Falkirk

CHATHAM – see Medway

69/1 **Chelmsford**, 12 Critchett Terrace, Primrose Hill, CM1 2QN 0245 357357

39/1 **Cheltenham**, 3 Clarence Road, Pittville, GL52 2AY 0242 515777

86/1 **Chester**, 36 Upper Northgate Street, CH1 4EF 0244 377999

154/1 **Chesterfield**, 2 Rose Hill, S40 1LW 0246 70000 & 204040

4/12 **Chicago**, IL, USA, 108 North State Street, Suite 1201, IL 60602 & 5638 S. Woodlawn Avenue, IL 60637 (The Society of Samaritans of Chicago) 312 947 8300

CHIENGMAYI, Thailand – in preparation

CHILTERNS – see Amersham

103A/1 **Cliftonville**, Caretaker's Flat, St Paul's Road, CT9 2DB (The Samaritans of Thanet, Associate Group of Canterbury q.v.) 0843 28877 (2 lines)

Coimbra, Portugal – in preparation

47/1 **Colchester**, 10 Vineyard Street, CO2 7DG 0206 561234

116/1 **Coleraine**, 20 Lodge Road, BT52 1NB 0265 4545

1/15 **Colombo 7**, Sri Lanka, Sri Lanka Sumithrayo, 60B Horton Place 92909

28/9 **Consolação**, São Paulo, SP Brazil, CVV-Samaritanos, Rua Nestor Pestana 136 terreo, CEP 01303 011 258 4111

COPACABANA – see Rio de Janeiro

125/1 **Cork**, Ireland, Coach Street 021 271323 (from London 010 353 21)

57/1 **Coventry**, 5a Priory Row, CV1 5EX 0203 225 50 & 24900

160/1 **Craigavon**, 162 Thomas Street, Portadown BT62 3BD 0762 333555

CRAWLEY – see Horsham

54/1 **Crewe**, 99 Edleston Road, CW2 7HP (The Samaritans of South Cheshire) 0270 216666

28/1 **Croydon**, 2B Kidderminster Road, CRO 2UE 681 6666/7/8

CUREPE – see Trinidad

16/9 **Curitiba**, PR, Brazil, CVV-Samaritanos, Rua Carneiro Lobo 35, Bairro Aqua Verde, CEP 80000 & Caixa Postal 7581 041 242 8811

92/1 **Darlington**, 13 Woodland Road, DL3 7BJ 0325 55353/4

DARTFORD – see Bexleyheath

8/1 **Derby**, 110 Burton Road, DE1 1TG 0332 364444/5

152/1 **Derry**, 16 Clarendon Street, BT48 7ET 0504 265511

56/9 **Diadema**, SP, Brazil, CVV-Samaritanos, Av Alda 56, Sala 2,3, CEP 09900 011 456 4111

33/1 **Doncaster**, 36 Thorne Road, DN1 2JA 0302 327474

DORSET – see Weymouth

172/1 **Douglas**, Isle of Man, 5 Victoria Place 0624 28211

110/1 **Dublin 2**, Ireland, 66 South William Street 778833 (UK code 0001)

176/1 **Dumfries**, Loreburn Hall, Newall Terrace, DG1 1LN 0387 53555

19/1 **Dundee**, 10 Victoria Chambers DD1 1JN 0382 26666/7

62/1 **Dunfermline**, 30 Maygate, KY12 7NS 0383 722222

122/1 **Durham**, 26 Sutton Street, DH1 4BW 0385 42727

128/1 **Ealing**, London, 26 Junction Road, W5 4XL 560 2345

63/1 **Eastbourne**, 27 Susans Road, BN21 3TW 0323 35555

2/13 EAST LONDON, Republic of South Africa – in abeyance

EAST SURREY and NORTH SUSSEX – see Reigate

2/1 **Edinburgh**, 54 Frederick Street, EH2 1LN 031 225 3333

141/1 **Elgin**, 29 Batchen Street, IV30 1BH 0343 3000

147/1 **Enfield**, Bounds Green, London, 40 Queens Road, N11 2QU (The Samaritans of Enfield-Haringey-Barnet) 889 6888

186/1 **Ennis**, Co. Clare, Ireland, Sunville, Kilrush Road 065 29777 (from London 010 353 65)

ESTORIL, Portugal – in preparation

42/1 **Exeter**, 2 Wynards, Magdalen Street, EX2 4HX 0392 39898/9

73/1 **Falkirk**, 2/4 Leslie Place, Kerse Lane, FK1 1RG (The Samaritans of Central Scotland) 0324 22066/7

9/12 **Fall River**, MA, USA, 386 Stanley Street, MA 02720 (The Samaritans of Fall River & New Bedford) 617 636 6111

2/12 **Falmouth**, MA, USA, POB 65, MA 02541 (The Samaritans on Cape Cod) 617 548 8900 & 759 2828 & 771 7770 & 255 1888

168/1 **Farnborough**, 16 Closeworth Road, GU14 6JH 0252 513222

149/1 FESTIVAL BRANCH (for Samaritan work in the open at Pop Festivals etc.) c/o 17 Uxbridge Road, Slough, SL1 1SN

43/1 **Folkestone**, 19 Cambridge Gardens, CT20 1OB 0303 55000

10/12 **Framingham**, MA, USA, 73 Union Street, MA 01701 (The Samaritans of South Middlesex) 617 875 4500

27/9 **Franca**, SP, Brazil, CVV-Samaritanos, Rua Nuno Alberto 1654, CEP 14400 & Caixa Postal 43 016 723 1444

167/1 **Galway**, Ireland, 14 Nun's Island (091) 61222 (from London 010 353 91)

1/8 **Gdańsk**, Poland, Anonimowy Przyjaciel, ul. Grodzka 20, 80-841

4/1 **Glasgow**, 218 West Regent Street, G2 4DQ 041 248 4488

121X/1 **Gloucester**, Basement, 1 Belgrave Road, GL1 1LT 0452 36333/4

15/9 **Goiânia**, Goiás, Brazil, CVV-Samaritanos, Rua 72, 277 Setor Central, CEP 74000 062 224 4048 & 233 4041

1/18 **Göteborg 41123**, Sweden, Nagon att tala med, Samaritans, Vastergatan 1A, 031 112400 & 112422

GOTHENBURG – see Göteborg

74B/1 **Grantham**, Town Hall, St Peter's Hill, NG31 6PY (Associate Group of Lincoln q.v.) 0476 67616

158/1 **Great Yarmouth**, 62 North Quay, NR30 1JB 0493 842800

5/6 GREYMOUTH S., New Zealand – in abeyance

56/1 **Grimsby**, 55 Alexandra Road, DN31 1RD 0472 53111/2

38/9 **Guarulhos**, SP, Brazil, CVV-Samaritanos, Rua 7 de Setembro 151 sala 35 CEP 07000 011 913 5781

30/1 **Guernsey**, CI, 2 Forest Lane, St Peter Port 0481 23731/2

34/1 **Guildford**, 69 Woodbridge Road, GU1 4RD 0483 505555

HAAD YAI, Thailand – in preparation

22/1 **Halifax**, Warwick Chambers, 37 Southgate, HX1 1DL 0422 58585/6

136/1 **Hamilton**, 4 Selkirk Place, ML3 6RQ 0698 429411

1/4 **Harare**, Zimbabwe, POB UA 267, Union Avenue 22000 & 20201

HARLOW – see Ware

162/1 **Harrogate**, 3 Mount Parade, HG1 1BX 0423 525 352

Harrow (Lond), 2 St John's Road, HA1 2HA 427 7777

12/12 **Hartford**, CT, USA, 646 Prospect Avenue, CT 06105 & POB 12004, CT 06112 (The Samaritans of the Capitol Region) 203 561 3610

111/1 **Hartlepool**, 58 Avenue Road, TS24 8AT 0429 272929 & 276767

38/1 **Hastings**, 26 St Andrew's Square, TN34 1SR (The Samaritans of Hastings and Rother) 0424 436666

179/1 **Haverfordwest**, 6 Tower Hill, SA61 2LJ 0437 5536 & 66699

HAVERING – see Romford

HEMEL HEMPSTEAD – see Watford

135/1 **Hereford**, 21 King Street, HR4 9BX 0432 269000

HERTS/ESSEX – see Ware

138/1 **Hillingdon**, 2 Press Road, Uxbridge UB8 1AT 0895 53355

146/1 **Hitchin**, 5 Nuns Close, SG5 1EP (The Samaritans of North Herts. & Stevenage) 0462 55333 (Hitchin) 0438 316161 (Stevenage)

2/2 **Hong Kong**, The Samaritans English Speaking Service, Sailors' and Soldiers' Home, 22 Hennessy Road 3rd floor, Wanchai 5-27 8484

140/1 **Horsham**, 21 Denne Road, RH12 1JE (The Samaritans of Horsham and Crawley) Horsham 0403 56111 Crawley 0293 34549

98/1 **Huddersfield**, 47 Trinity Street, HD1 4DN 0484 533388/9

14/1 **Hull**, 75 Spring Bank, HU3 1AG 0482 23456

4/6 **Hutt Valley**, 42 Laings Road, Lower Hutt & POB 30388 Wellington N. 664 591

81/1 **Ilford**, 8 Mildmay Road, IG1 1DZ (The Samaritans of Redbridge) 478 7273

142/1 **Inverness**, 66 Tomnahurich Street, IV3 5DT 0463 234000

2/11 **Ipoh**, West Malaysia, The Befrienders, Servants' Quarters, behind the Anglican Church & POB 413 05 540559 & 543435 (4 pm to midnight)

29/1 **Ipswich**, 19 Tower Street, IP1 3BE 0473 211133

ISLE OF MAN – see Douglas

ISLE OF WIGHT (Associate Group of Portsmouth, q.v.) 14 East Street, Newport PO30 1JL 0983 521234

43/9 **Jaboticabal**, SP, Brazil, CVV-Samaritanos, Av. General Glicerio 509 CEP 14870 0163 220005

1/42 **Jakarta**, Indonesia, Dharma Samaritan, Hotline Service Bersama, POB 96/KBYB, Jakarta 12001, Selantan 771810 & 733399

11/1 **Jersey**, CI, 30 Hue Street, St Helier 0534 25555/6

4/9 **Jundiai**, SP, Brazil, CVV-Samaritanos, Rua Visconde de Maua 174, Vila Municipal, CEP 13200 011 434 4037 & 4141

3/7 **Kalgoorlie**, Western Australia 6430, POB 480 090 21 4111

2/15 **Kandy**, Sri Lanka, Sri Lanka Sumithrayo, YMCA Building, Sangaraja Mawatha

5/12 **Keene**, NH, USA, 25 Lamson Street, NH 03431 603 357 5505

95A/1 **Kettering**, (Associate Group of Northampton, q.v.) 123 Montagu Street, NN16 8XL 0536 516333

70/1 **Kilmarnock**, 43 Titchfield Street, KA1 1QS (The Samaritans of Kilmarnock and Ayrshire) 0563 31313

3/13 **Kimberley**, 8300 RSA, Red Cross House, Stockdale Street, 8301 & POB 38, 8300 0531 23313

153/1 **Kings Lynn**, 26 Queen Street, PE30 1HT 0553 761616 & 761617

97/1 **Kingston on Thames**, 12 St Andrew's Road, Surbiton, KT6 4DT 399 6676/7/8

164/1 **Kirkcaldy**, 50 Rosslyn Street, KY1 3AB 0592 265444

2/14 KITWE, Zambia – in abeyance

1/11 **Kuala Lumpur**, West Malaysia, The Befrienders, 95 Jalan Templer, Petaling Jaya, Selangor

1/43 LAGOS, Nigeria – in preparation.

132/1 **Lancaster**, 21 Sun Street, LA1 1EW 0524 61666

LAPA – see Rio de Janeiro

4/7 **Launceston**, Tasmania, Australia 7250, Life Link, POB 228 31 3355

6/12 **Lawrence**, MA, USA, 55 Jackson Street, MA 01840 (The Samaritans of Merrimack Valley) 617 688 6607 (Lawrence) & 452 6733 (Lowell) & 372 7200 (Haverhill)

58/1 **Leatherhead**, 7 Church Road, KT22 8AT 0372 375555

79/1 **Leeds**, 93 Clarendon Road, LS2 9LY 0532 456789

65/1 **Leek**, 34 Fountain Street, ST13 6JR 0538 384100

44/1 **Leicester**, la Elmfield Avenue, LE2 1RB 0533 700007

LERWICK – see Shetland

2/36 **Lethbridge**, Alberta, Canada, 1256 Sixth Avenue South T1J 1A4 403 320 1212 & 9334; also (no toll charge) Zenith 66003

100/1 **Lewisham**, 362 New Cross Road, London SE14 6AG 692 5228

LEYTON – see Waltham Forest

25/9 **Limeira**, SP, Brazil, CVV-Samaritanos, Rua Boa Morte 1075, CEP 13480 0194 41 0147 & 6439

159/1 **Limerick**, Ireland, 25 Upper Cecil Street (061) 42111 (from London 010 353 61)

74/1 **Lincoln**, 17 Hungate, LN1 1ES 0522 28282

37/9 **Lins**, SP, Brazil, CVV-Samaritanos, Rua Voluntario Vitoriano Borges 430 fundos, CEP 16400 0145 22 2022

3/1 **Liverpool**, 25 Clarence Street, L3 5TN (The Samaritans of Liverpool and Merseyside) 051 708 8888

1/1 **London**, 39 Walbrook, EC4N 8BP and 3 Hornton Place, W8 4LZ (The Samaritans, Central London Branch) (tubes, Bank or Cannon Street & High Street Kensington) 283 3400 NB Move to new premises planned in 1987.
Other Branches in London are Bexley & Dartford, Brent, Croydon, Ealing, Enfield-Haringey-Barnet, Harrow, Havering, Hillingdon, Kingston, Lewisham, Orpington, Putney, Redbridge and Watford.

LONDONDERRY – see Derry

36/9 **Londrina**, PR, Brazil, CVV-Samaritanos, Praca 1 de Maia S/No & Caixa Postal 2132, CEP 86100 0432 22 3432

34/9 **Lorena**, SP, Brazil, CVV-Samaritanos, Rua Comendador Custodio Ferreira 339 & Caixa Postal 145 52 11 55

LOWER HUTT – see Hutt Valley

120/1 **Lowestoft**, 14 Beach Road, NR32 1EA (The Samaritans of Lowestoft & Waveney) 0502 2800 & 3313

77/1 **Luton**, 32 Napier Road, LU1 1RF 0582 20666

80/1 **Macclesfield**, 1–3 Exchange Street East, SK11 6LW 0625 27000 & 26000

6/3 **Madras**, India, Sneha, 4 Lloyds Lane, Roya Pettah

MAIDENHEAD – see Slough

157/1 **Maidstone**, 48 Grecian Street, ME14 2TS 0622 674444/5

7/1 **Manchester**, 87 Oldham Street, M4 1LN 061 834 9000

13/12 **Manchester**, NH, USA, (The Samaritans of South Central New Hampshire), 2013 Elm Street, NH 03103

1/45 **Manila**, Philippines – in preparation. Correspondent: Dr V.S. Cabuquit, MD, DPM, UERM Hospital, Aurora Blvd., Quezon City.

126/1 **Mansfield**, la Grove Street, NG18 1EL 0623 31515/6

1/21 **Mar del Plata 7600**, Argentina, CVV-Samaritanos, Galeria de las Americas, San Martin 2648 local 48 30 430

MARGATE – see Cliftonville

53/9 **Marilia**, SP, Brazil, CVV-Samaritanos, Rua 24 de Dezembro 1251 sala 11 CEP17500 0144 331677

7/4 **Marondera**, Zimbabwe, 40 Fourth Street (Associate Group of Harare, q.v.)

MARTHA'S VINEYARD – Associate Group of Falmouth, q.v.

3/6 **Masterton**, New Zealand, (The Samaritans of Wairarapa), YMCA Premises, Church Street & POB 366 81259

19/9 **Matarazzo**, São Paulo, SP, Brazil, CVV-Samaritanos, Alameda Rio Claro 190, J. Paulista, CEP 01332 011 289 4111 & 4133

57/9 **Maua**, SP, Brazil, CVV-Samaritanos, Av. Capitao Joao 300, Centro, CEP 09300 450 4111

MEDWAY – see Rochester

MERSEYSIDE – see Liverpool

1/37 **Mexico City**, DF, Mexico, Los Samaritanos, Rio Panuco 15, Col. Cuauhtemoc & POB 41 659 ZP 06500 566 3957 & 566 3997

96/1 **Middlesbrough**, 147 Borough Road, TS1 3AT (The Samaritans of Teesside) 0642 217777

MILLIWACH, BC, Canada – in preparation

180/1 **Milton Keynes**, 161 Fishermead Boulevard, Fishermead, MK6 2AB 0908 667777

42/9 **Mogi das Cruzes**, SP, Brazil, CVV-Samaritanos, Caixa Postal 214, CEP 08700 469 6444

1/24 **Montevideo**, Uruguay, CVV-Samaritanos, 8 de Octubre 3324 70 10 24

1/44 **Muscat** – The Befrienders, POB 4982, Ruwi, Sultanate of Oman 799474

3/4 **Mutare**, Zimbabwe, 121 First Street & POB 133 63559

1/46 NAIROBI, Kenya – in preparation

31/9 **Natal**, RN, Brazil, CVV-Samaritanos, Rua João Pessoa 219, Ed. Sisal s.602, CEP 59000 084 222 0226

1/23 **Neiva-Huila**, Colombia, CVV-Samaritanos, Calle 47 no. 1-A-52 & Apdo. Aereo 495 46185 & 47723

NELSON – see Pendle

NEW BEDFORD – see Fall River

24A/1 **Newbury** (Associate Group of Reading, q.v.) Sterling Industrial Estate, King's Road, RG14 5RA 0635 42452

67/1 **Newcastle**, 24 Portland Terrace, NE2 1QS (The Samaritans of Tyneside) 091 2327272

90/1 **Newport**, 43 Stow Hill, NP9 1JH (The Samaritans of Newport & Gwent) 0633 59000

144/1 **Newry**, Co. Down, 11 Lower Catherine Street, BT35 6BE 0693 66366

7/12 **New York City**, NY, USA, 61 Gramercy Park North, 6th fl., NY 10010 212 673 3000 & 664 0505

59/1 **Northallerton**, 7 Crosby Road, DL6 1AA (The Samaritans of Northallerton & The Dales) 0609 6161

95/1 **Northampton**, 2 St Michael's Avenue, NN1 4JQ 0604 20241

NORTH DEVON – see Barnstaple

NORTH HERTS – see Hitchin

NORTH SUSSEX and EAST SURREY – see Reigate

78/1 **Northwich**, 1 St Paul's Place, Witton Street, CW9 5DZ (The Samaritans of Mid-Cheshire) 0606 3211/2

46/1 **Norwich**, 19 St Stephen's Square, NR1 3SS 0603 611311

18/1 **Nottingham**, 18 Clarendon Street, NG1 5HQ 0602 411111

161/1 **Omagh**, Co. Tyrone, 20 Campsie Road, BT37 0AB 0662 44944/5

1/30 **Oporto**, Portugal, Telefone de Amizade, Apartado 606, 4010 Porto Codex 672727

71/1 **Orpington**, 9b Station Road, BR6 0RZ 0689 33000 & 33999

1/25 **Osaka 542**, Japan, Suicide Prevention, 38 Sennen-cho, Minami-ku 06 251 4343 & 4339

45/9 **Osasco**, São Paulo, SP, Brazil, CVV-Samaritanos, Rue Tenente Avelar Pires de Azevedo 396 CEP 0600 011 803 1111

32/1 **Oxford**, 123 Iffley Road, OX4 1EJ 0865 722122

2/6 **Palmerston N.**, New Zealand, (The Samaritans of Manawatu) 15 Amesbury Street & POB 1963 744 00

39/9 **Paraiba**, SP, Brazil, CVV-Samaritanos, Av. Manuel Deodato 886 083 224 4726

1/27 PARAMARIBO, Surinam – in abeyance

1/16 **Paris**, France, SOS-Help, St George's Church, Rue Auguste Vacquerie, Boîte Postale 239.16, 75765 Paris Cedex 16 723 8080

3/11 **Penang**, Malaysia, The Befrienders, Counselling Centre, Wisma Pengakap, 1 Scotland Close 682233 & 688977

151/1 **Pendle**, 15 Market Square, Nelson, BB9 7LP (The Samaritans of Pendle & Burnley) 0282 694929

113/1 **Perth**, 59 King Street, PH2 8SB 0738 26666

1/7 **Perth**, Western Australia, 60 Bagot Road, Subiaco 6008 09 381 5555 & 5725 (Samaritan Youth Line, same address, 381 2500)

PETALING JAYA – see Kuala Lumpur

119/1 **Peterborough**, 41 Eastfield Road, PE1 4AP 0733 64848 & 48222

3/36 **Pincher Creek**, Alberta, Canada, POB 2455, T4C 1WO

5/9 **Pinheiros**, São Paulo, SP, Brazil, CVV-Samaritanos, Henrique Schaumann 163, CEP 05413 011 883 4111

29/9 **Piracicaba**, SP, Brazil, CVV-Samaritanos, Rue Regente Feijo 1036, CEP 13400 0194 332908

134/1 **Plymouth**, 20 Oxford Place, PL1 5AJ 0752 221666

6/7 PORT HEDLAND – temporarily in abetance

PORTO – see Oporto

2/9 **Porto Alegre**, Brazil: the three Branches are no longer affiliated to CVV-Samaritanos, but to Amigos Anônimos, also part of B.I., Av. Oswaldo Aranha, 1092 conj. 07, CEP 90000 25 0612

58/9 **Porto Alegre 2**, Pronto Socorro Municipal, CEP 90000 25 0612

59/9 **Porto Alegre 3**, Av. de Acesso, S/N, Vila Mapa, CEP 90000 25 0612

PORT OF SPAIN – see Trinidad

17/1 **Portsmouth**, 296 London Road, North End, PO2 9JN (The Samaritans of Portsmouth District and Isle of Wight) 0705 691313/4/5

1/31 PORT VILA, Vanuatu – in abeyance

40/9 **Presidente Prudente**, SP, Brazil, CVV-Samaritanos, Av. Washington Luiz 874, 2 Andar, CEP 19100 0182 33 5157

51/9 **Presidente Wenceslau**, SP, Brazil, CVV-Samaritanos, Praca Santo Antonio S/N, CEP 19400 0182 71 2231

109/1 **Preston**, 11 St Wilfred Street, PR1 2US 0772 22022

3/12 **Providence**, RI, USA, 33 Chestnut Street, RI 02903 401 2724044

123/1 **Putney**, London, 106 Felsham Road, SW15 1DQ 789 9121/2

24/1 **Reading**, 154 Southampton Street, RG1 2RD 0734 54845

9/9 **Recife**, PE, Brazil, CVV-Samaritanos, Travessa Barão de São Borja 44, Bairro Boa Vista, CEP 50000 081 231 4141

REDBRIDGE – see Ilford

53/1 **Reigate**, 4b High Street, RH2 9AY (The Samaritans of East Surrey) 073 72 48444/5

74C/1 **Retford**, The Wharf (next to Fire Station), Carolgate, DN22 6EN (Associate Group of Lincoln, q.v.) 0777 703939

145/1 **Rhyl**, 23 Bedford Street, LL18 1SY (The Samaritans of Clwyd & Gwynedd) 0745 54545

23/9 **Riberão Preto**, SP, Brazil, CVV-Samaritanos, Rua Lafayette 1071, CEP 14100 016 636 5623 & 5626

10/9 **Rio de Janeiro**, RJ, Brazil, CVV-Samaritanos, Avenida Rio Branco 156, sala 720, CEP 20040 021 262 4141

49/9 **Rio de Janeiro**, RJ, Brazil, CVV-Samaritanos Copacabana, Av. N. Sra. Copacabana 435, sala 908, CEP 22020 021 256 4141

44/9 **Rio de Janeiro**, RJ, Brazil, CVV-Samaritanos Lapa, Rua Teotonio Regadas 26, sala 504, CEP 20021 021 242 9292

13/9 **Rio de Janeiro**, RJ, Brazil, CVV-Samaritanos Tijuca, Rua General Roca 158, Casa no. 1, CEP 20521 021 254 9191 & 9393

83/1 **Rochdale**, 4 Oldham Road, OL11 1BU 0706 59998

76/1 **Rochester**, 42 Ross Street, ME1 2DF (The Samaritans of Medway) 0634 44846 & 42222

1/32 **Rome**, Italy, San Silvestro in Capite, Piazza San Silvestro 8, 00187 (near GPO) 6789 227

64/1 **Romford**, 107 North Street, RM1 1ER (The Samaritans of Havering) 0708 751111 & 40000

177/1 **Rotherham**, 22 Percy Street, S65 1ED 0709 361717

7/6 **Rotorua**, New Zealand, Life Link & Youthline, Contact House, Cnr. of Fenton and Arawa Streets & POB 1682 06473 80567

8/12 **Salem**, MA, USA, 90 Highland Avenue & POB 8133, MA 01971 (The Samaritans of the North Shore) 617 744 5000

26/1 **Salisbury**, 42 Milford Street, SP1 2BP 0722 23355

63/9 SANTA BARBARA, SP, Brazil – in preparation. Correspondent: A. J. B. Quirino, R. Dna. Margarida 1477, CEP 13458 0194 63 1561

64/9 SANTA CATARINA, Brazil – in preparation. Correspondent: A. D. Bordin, R. Cons. Mafra 40, s. 803, CEP 88000

1/33 SANTIAGO, Chile – in preparation. Correspondent: Sra. Paz Betancourt Johnson, Los Diamelos 2911, 5. 9

41/9 **Santo Amaro**, São Paulo, SP, Brazil, CVV-Samaritanos, Av. Adolfo Pinheiro 805, CEP 04733 011 247 4111 (if no answer ring Barra Funda)

3/9 **Santo André**, SP, Brazil, CVV-Samaritanos, Rua Dr Cesario Motta 27, CEP 090000 011 449 4111

18/9 **Santos**, Av. Francisco Manoel S/N 0132 34 4111

35/9 **São Bernardo do Campo**, SP, Brazil, CVV-Samaritanos, Rua Joachim Nabuco 380, CEP 09710 011 443 4141

20/9 **São Caetano do Sul**, SP, Brazil, CVV-Samaritanos, Rua Monte Alegre 227, CEP 09500 011 744 4111

54/9 **São Carlos**, SP, Brazil, CVV-Samaritanos, Rua Gen. Osorio 575 Sala 01 0162 724111

26/9 **São José do Rio Preto**, SP, Brazil CVV-Samaritanos, Av. Alberto Andalo 3033, Centro, CEP 15100 0172 21 4442

6/9 **São José dos Campos**. SP, Brazil, CVV-Samaritanos, Av. Marechal Floriano Peixoto 180 salas 3 & 4, CEP 12200 0123 21 4111

1/9 **São Paulo**, SP, Brazil – see Abolição. Other Branches in Greater São Paulo are in Barra Funda, Consolação, Matarazzo, Osasco, Pinheiros, Santo Amaro, São Caetano, Tatuapé, Tatuapé 2, Vila Carrão, Vila Maria and Vila Mariana.
The administrative office for CVV-Samaritanos Brazil is at 168 Rue Genebra, CEP 01316, São Paulo, SP, Telex 011 21457, Tel. 32 3965 1–6 p.m.

61/9 **São Vicente**, SP, Brazil, CVV-Samaritanos, Av. Pres. Wilson 1473, CEP 11300 68 97 42

148/1 **Scarborough**, 35a St Nicholas Cliff, YO11 2ES 0723 368888

130/1 SCOTTISH CORRESPONDENCE BRANCH, POB 9, Stirling, FK8 2SA

49/1 **Scunthorpe**, Lyndum House, 2 Lindum Street, DN15 6QU 0724 860000

178/1 **Selkirk**, Kirk Wynd (The Samaritans of The Borders) 0750 2000

1/41 **Seoul**, Korea, Love Line, Social Welfare Building, 427–5 Kong Duk Dong, Mapo-ku 714 0770

61/1 **Sheffield**, 30 Rockingham Lane, S1 4FW 0742 767277

SHERBORNE – see Yeovil

185/1 **Shetland Islands**, 26 North Road, Lerwick ZE1 0PQ 0595 4449

51/1 **Shrewsbury**, 14 Castle Court, SY1 2AJ 0743 69696/7

60/9 **Silvio Romero**, SP, Brazil, CVV-Samaritanos, Rua Isidro Tinoco 111, CEP 04012 011 293 4111

183/1 **Sligo**, Republic of Ireland, 12 Chapel Street (from UK: 0103 5371) 42011/2

102/1 **Slough**, Tregantle, 10 Ledgers Road, SL1 2QX (The Samaritans of Slough, Windsor & Maidenhead) 0753 31011 (NB Not to be confused with the General Office of The Samaritans Inc. at 17 Uxbridge Road, Slough SL1 1SN)

150/1 **Solihull**, Station Approach, B91 1LE 021 704 2255

46/9 **Sorocaba**, SP, Brazil, CVV-Samaritanos, Fundacão Ubaldino Amaral, Rue Miranda Azevedo 464, CEP 18100 0152 31 4946 & 4614

35/1 **Southampton**, 64/5 St Andrew's Road, SO2 0BA 0703 32888/9

75/1 **Southend on Sea**, 54 Hamlet Road, SS1 1HH 0702 333999

170/1 **Southport**, 32 Union Street, PR9 0QE 0704 38038

8/7 **Springwood**, N.S.W., Australia, The Samaritans, Befrienders and Carers Group, Civic Centre Complex, & P.O. Box 161, Springwood 2777 (047) 51 3033

40/1 **Stafford**, Chell Road, ST16 2QA 0785 43333 (2 lines)

STEVENAGE – see Hitchin

STIRLING – see Scottish Correspondence Branch

7A/1 **Stockport**, Churchgate House, 96 Churchgate SK1 1YJ (Associate Group of Manchester) 061 480 2222

STOCKTON – see Teesside

21/1 **Stoke on Trent**, 3 Shelton New Road, Shelton, ST1 4PF (The Samaritans of Stoke on Trent & Newcastle District) 0782 23555

108/1 **Sunderland**, 13 Grange Crescent, SR2 7BN 0783 77177

1/34 SUVA, Fiji – in preparation

16/1 **Swansea**, 5 Willows Place, SA1 6AA 0792 55999

91/1 **Swindon**, 5/6 Curtis Street, SN1 5JU 0793 37373

25A/1 **Tamworth**, 1a King Street, B79 7DB (Associate Group of Birmingham, q.v.) 0827 54222

11/9 **Tatuapé**, São Paulo, SP, Brazil, CVV-Samaritanos, Rua Siria 67, CEP 03086 011 941 4111

12/9 **Taubaté**, SP, Brazil, CVV-Samaritanos, Rua Dr Barbosa de Oliveira S/N, CEP 12100 0122 31 4111

6/6 **Tauranga**, New Zealand, 14 Hamilton Street & POB Brooklyn 6309 81001

94/1 **Taunton**, 16 Wood Street, TA1 1UN (The Samaritans of Taunton & Somerset) 0823 88998/9

TEESSIDE – see Middlesborough

156/1 **Telford**, 115 King Street, Wellington, TF1 1NU 0952 56161/2

THANET – see Cliftonville

187/1 **Thurso**, 7 Riverside Place, Highland Region of Scotland KW14 8BZ (The Samaritans of Caithness) 0847 5656

TIJUCA – see Rio de Janeiro

TORBAY – see Torquay

55/1 **Torquay**, 21 Warren Road, TQ2 5TQ (The Samaritans of South Devon) 0803 25355

1/22 **Trinidad**, West Indies, Lifeline (The Befrienders of Trinidad & Tobago) Corner of Francis & Sellier Streets, Curepe & POB 1224 Port of Spain 662 5178

4/3 **Trivandrum 695014**, Kerala, India, The Samaritans, 'Harshini', TC no. 15/1082, Voltas Lane, Vazhuthacaud, Kerala

114/1 **Truro**, 19 Treyew Road, TR1 2BY 0872 77277

85/1 **Tunbridge Wells**, 7 Lime Hill Road, TN1 1LJ 0892 32323

TYNESIDE – see Newcastle

59/9 **Uberaba**, M. G., Brazil, CVV-Samaritanos, Rua Artur Machado 76, s. 205–7, CEP 38100 034 333 5353

UMTALI – see Mutare

UXBRIDGE – see Hillingdon

1/19 **Vienna 1030**, Austria, The Befrienders, Seidlgasse 8/3 73 33 74

50/9 **Vila Carrão**, São Paulo, SP, Brazil, CVV-Samaritanos, Av. Guilherme Cotching 1219, Apto. 12, CEP 02113 011 264 4311

47/9 **Vila Maria**, São Paulo, SP, Brazil, CVV-Samaritanos, Av. Guilherme Cotching 1219, Apto. 12, CEP 02113 011 264 4311

48/9 **Vila Mariana**, São Paulo, SP, Brazil, CVV-Samaritanos, Rua Domingos de Morães 348, Galeria Capri sala 34, CEP 04010 011 575 4111

62/9 **Vitoria**, ES, Brazil, CVV-Samaritanos, Rua Sete de Setembro 530, CEP 29000 027 223 4111

124/1 **Wakefield**, 1/3 Jacob's Well Lane, WF1 3NN 0924 377011

106/1 **Walsall**, Bott Lane, WS1 2JQ 0922 24000 & 20000

81A/1 **Waltham Forest**, 633 Lea Bridge Road, Leyton E10 9BY (Associate Group of Redbridge, see Ilford) 01-520 1181

WANCHAI – see Hong Kong

8/6 **Wanganui**, New Zealand, 120 Guyton Street & Box 4116 Mid-Avenue PO 55090

10/1 **Ware**, 14 Cross Street, SG12 7AH (The Samaritans of Herts/Essex) 0920 4099 & Welwyn Garden 32222, & Harlow 21110

104/1 **Warrington**, 46 Arpley Street, WA1 1LX 0925 38808/9

15/12 **Washington**, DC, USA, – in abeyance

166/1 **Waterford**, Ireland, 13 Beau Street (051) 72114 (from London 010 353 51)

107/1 **Watford**, 2 Local Board Road, WD1 1LJ (The Samaritans of South West Herts) 0923 33333

WELLINGTON – see Telford

1/6 **Wellington N.**, New Zealand, Cathedral Building, Molesworth Street & POB 12044 739739

WELWYN GARDEN CITY – see Ware

184/1 **Weston super Mare**, 137a High Street, BS23 1HN 0934 32555

50/1 **Weybridge**, Samaritan Centre, Ledger Drive, Addlestone, KT15 1AT (The Samaritans of North West Surrey) 0932 44444 & 46444

117/1 **Weymouth**, 13 King Street, DT4 7BJ (The Samaritans of Dorset) 030 57 771777/8

84/1 **Whitehaven**, 49 Duke Street, CA28 7NU (The Samaritans of West Cumbria) 0946 4266

127/1 **Wigan**, 73 Dicconson Street, WN1 2AT 0942 492222

165/1 **Winchester**, 10 Parchment Street, SO22 6RN 0962 60633

WINDSOR – see Slough

153A/1 **Wisbech**, 63 Lynn Road, PI3 7DE (Associate Group of King's Lynn q.v.) 0945 61616/7

60/1 **Wolverhampton**, 54 Newhampton Road West, WV6 0RU 0902 26422/3

WOLVERTON – see Milton Keynes

36/1 **Worcester**, 9 Sansome Place, WR1 1UA 0905 21121

61A/1 **Worksop**, Samaritan House, 71 Eastgate, S80 1RE (Associate Group of Sheffield q.v.) 0909 486345

101/1 **Worthing**, 2 Lennox Road, BN11 1DA 0903 205555/6

129/1 **Yeovil**, 10 Everton Road, BA20 1UF 0935 76455 & 23466

89/1 **York**, 89 Nunnery Lane, YO2 1AH 0904 55888/9

Useful addresses

The Samaritans

ROYAL PATRON	HRH The Duchess of Kent
CHAIRMAN	The Revd Albert Jewell, 54 Whitecote Hill, Bramley, Leeds, LS13 2HU
VICE-CHAIRMEN	Dr Norman Keir, Teesside Branch Mrs Elizabeth Reeve, Tunbridge Wells Branch Miss Kathy Biggar, Central London Branch

Regional representatives

IRELAND	Mr Roger Byers, Dublin Branch
SCOTLAND	Mr Bob Clark, Hamilton Branch
NORTH WEST	Mrs Joan Guénault, Lancaster Branch
NORTH	Mrs Sheila Coggrave, Sunderland Branch
NORTH EAST	Mr Kenneth Chilvers, Huddersfield Branch
WEST MIDLANDS & NORTH WALES	Mr Keith Greenaway, Walsall Branch
EAST MIDLANDS	Mr Maurice Walton Northampton Branch
EAST	Mrs Sarah Sherwood, Colchester Branch

LONDON	Dr Alan Isaacs, Harrow Branch
SOUTH EAST	Mrs Dorothy Lewis, Leatherhead Branch
SOUTH	Mrs Daphne Minihane, Jersey Branch
SOUTH WALES & THE MARCHES	Mr Julian Hughes, Cardiff Branch
SOUTH WEST	Dr Christine Hall, Exeter Branch
HON. SOLICITOR	Mr Michael Charman, 10 New Street, Leicester, LE1 5ND
HON. PUBLICITY OFFICER	Mr Rex Cannon, 45 Boundstone Road, Boundstone, Farnham, Surrey, GU10 4TW Telephone: Frensham 2085 (025 125)
HON. BURSAR	Mr James Wheeler, Stocks Mead, Arkesden, Saffron Walden, Essex, CB11 4EY
HON. YOUTH OFFICER	Mr Nick Ellerby, Hull Branch
GENERAL SECRETARY	The Revd David Evans, 17 Uxbridge Road, Slough, SL1 1SN Telephone: Slough 32713 (0753)
ASST. GEN. SECRETARY	Mr Simon Armson, 17 Uxbridge Road, Slough, SL1 1SN
APPEALS DIRECTOR	Mrs Valerie Pakenham Keady, Samaritan Campaign Office, 3 Hornton Place, London, W8 4LZ Telephone 01-937 2537
SAMARITAN BOOKS (Ken & Chris)	110 Burton Road, Derby, DE1 1TG
SAMARITAN MAGAZINE	Ms Elisabeth Salisbury, 88 Kendrick Road, Reading, Berks, RG1 5DN

The Samaritans: Befriending the suicidal

SAMARITAN TAPES *(Cheques made payable to 'The Samaritans')*	Richard and Moyra Montagu, 6 Fleur Gates, Princes Way, London, SW19 6QQ Telephone 01-788 4224 (All orders and enquiries to the above address)
SAMARITAN FILM 'Can I Help You?' (16 mm, colour & sound)	The Samaritans, 17 Uxbridge Road, Slough, SL1 1SN

Befrienders International (The Samaritans Worldwide)

CHAIRMAN	Mrs Vanda Scott, PO Box 50029 Dallas, TX 75250, USA Telephone: 214 243 6110
SECRETARY	Mrs Anne Aston, (Also Editor of Befriending Worldwide) 40 Andrew Road Singapore 1129

Continental Representatives

AFRICA	Mrs Pam Williams, POB 2201, Bloemfontein 9301, Rep. of South Africa
AMERICA CENTRAL AND SOUTH	(vacant)
AMERICA NORTH	Mrs Karin Bohr, 55 Jackson Street, MA 01840, USA
ASIA EAST	Miss Tan Yoke-Sim, POB 413, Ipoh, Malaysia

ASIA WEST	Mrs Kiran S. Bhatia, C 4/69 S D Area, New Delhi 110 016, India
AUSTRALASIA AND OCEANIA	Mrs Charlotte Keay, 60 Bagot Road, Subiaco 6008, Western Australia
EUROPE	Fru Greta Meyersberg, Kungälvsgatan 8 B, 41669 Göteborg, Sweden

National representatives

BRAZIL	Senhor Eduardo Ossege, SDS Ed. Venancio IV, Sala 311, CEP 70300 Brasilia DF
NEW ZEALAND	Mr Brian Moffitt, Chairman, BINZ, 66 Bloomfield Terrace, Lower Hutt, New Zealand
USA	Mrs Karin Bohr, 55 Jackson Street, MA 01840, USA
ZIMBABWE	Mr Pieter De Bruijn, National Council of Samaritans, PO Box UA267, Harare Zimbabwe
CONSULTANT	(Liaison with The Samaritans) Mrs Loveday Russell, The Briars, Cliff Road, Hythe, Kent, CT21 5XQ, UK
HON. LAWYER	Mr Mike Charman, 10 New Street, Leicester, LE1 5ND, UK

List of contributors

DOMINIQUE ALESSANDRI is a Psychiatrist in Lyons, and a member of Groupement d'Etudes et Prévention du Suicide

CHARLES BAGG, MA, MRCS, LRCP, MRCPsych, DPM was a Consultant Psychiatrist until his retirement

J. L. T. BIRLEY, FRCP, FRCPsych is Dean of Psychiatry at the Maudsley Hospital, London, and Consultant Psychiatrist to The Samaritans (Inc.)

BELA BUDA, MD, is a Hungarian Psychiatrist and Suicidologist

REX CANNON is Honorary Publicity Officer of The Samaritans (Inc.) and a Samaritan volunteer

SALLY CASPER is a former Director of The Samaritans of Merrimack Valley, MA, USA

The late DAVID DAVIES, DM (Oxon), FRCP, FRCPsych was Medical Director of the Alcohol Education Centre at the Maudsley Hospital, London

GEORGE DAY, MA, MD is a Consultant to The Samaritans (Inc.)

CAROLINE BENEDICT DREW is a former Director of The Samaritans of Providence, RI, USA

JOHN ELDRID, AKC is Director of the Central London Branch of The Samaritans, and a former Chairman of The Samaritans (Inc.)

BARBARA ESPEY is a former President of The Samaritans USA and SW (BI) representative for America North

ROSEMARY HANSON is a Samaritan volunteer

DAVID HOGARTH is Director of Lifeline attached to The Samaritans of Boston, MA, USA

PETER M. JEFFERYS, MA, MB, BCh, MRCP, FRCPsych, is a Consultant Psychiatrist at Northwick Park Hospital, Harrow, Middlesex

NUALA KELLY is a Samaritan volunteer

P. W. W. LEACH, MB, ChB is a Consultant Psychiatrist

EMILY MEIR, MA(Oxon), SRN, RMN, RNJ, STh, was a Ward Sister at the Maudsley Hospital London and later Matron of The Priory, Roehampton, London

IVOR H. MILLS, PhD, MD, FRCP, Hon. FACP is Professor of Medicine in the University of Cambridge

The late DORIS ODLUM, MA, FRCPsych, DPM was for many years Consultant Psychiatrist to, and later President of, The Samaritans

COLIN MURRAY PARKES, MD, MRCPsych is an Honorary Consultant Psychiatrist

KENNETH RAWNSLEY, MB, ChB, FRCP, DPM is Professor of Psychiatry in the University of Wales College of Medicine

The late W. LINFORD REES, MD. BSc, FRCP, DPM was Professor of Psychiatry at St Bartholomew's Hospital, London

WILLIAM SARGANT, MA, MD, FRCP, DPM is a Consultant Psychiatrist at St Thomas' Hospital, London

VANDA SCOTT is Chairman of Befrienders International (The Samaritans Worldwide) and a former Director of The Samaritans of Wanchai, Hong Kong.

EDWIN S. SHNEIDMAN, PhD, is currently Professor of Thanatology in the University of California at Los Angeles. He is the recent author of *Definition of Suicide* (NY: Wiley, 1985)

GEORGE SPAUL, MB, BSc(Lond), MRCPsych, DPM is a Consultant Psychiatrist

ROY VINING, MB, BS is a medical practitioner and a Samaritan volunteer

H. J. WALTON, MB, PhD, FRCP, FRCPsych, DPM is Professor of Psychiatry at the University of Edinburgh

Editor

CHAD VARAH, OBE, MA(Oxon), Hon.LLD(Leicester), Honorary Fellow of Keble College Oxford is Rector of St Stephen Walbrook in the City of London, a Prebendary of St Paul's Cathedral, Founder of The Samaritans, holder of the Albert Schweitzer Gold Medal, the Louis I. Dublin Award of the American Association of Suicidology and the Prix de l'Institut de la Vie